ISO 9001:2000

A New Paradigm for Healthcare

Also available from ASQ Quality Press:

Improving Healthcare with Control Charts: Basic and Advanced SPC Methods and Case Studies
Raymond G. Carey

Accountability through Measurement: A Global Healthcare Imperative
Vahé A. Kazandjian

Measuring Quality Improvement in Healthcare: A Guide to Statistical Process Control Applications
Raymond G. Carey and Robert C. Lloyd

Customer Driven Healthcare: QFD for Process Improvement and Cost Reduction
Ed Chaplin and John Terninko

How to Use Patient Satisfaction Data to Improve Healthcare Quality
Ralph Bell and Michael Krivich

Nan: A Six Sigma Mystery
Robert Barry

To request a complimentary catalog of ASQ Quality Press publications, call 800-248-1946, or visit our Web site at http://qualitypress.asq.org.

ISO 9001:2000

A New Paradigm
for Healthcare

Bryce E. Carson, Sr.

ASQ Quality Press
Milwaukee, Wisconsin

American Society for Quality, Quality Press, Milwaukee 53203
© 2004 by ASQ
All rights reserved. Published 2003
Printed in the United States of America

12 11 10 09 08 07 06 05 04 03   5 4 3 2 1

Library of Congress Cataloging-in-Publication Data

Carson, Bryce E.
    ISO 9001:2000—a new paradigm for healthcare / Bryce E. Carson, Sr.
    p. cm.
    Includes bibliographical references and index.
    ISBN 0-87389-608-4 (softcover, casebound : alk. paper)
    1. Medical care—Standards. 2. Medical care—Quality control. 3. ISO
9000 Series Standards. I. Title.

RA399.A1C374 2003
362.1'02'18—dc22   2003024541

ISBN 0-87389-608-4

Publisher: William A. Tony
Acquisitions Editor: Annemieke Hytinen
Project Editor: Paul O'Mara
Production Administrator: Randy Benson
Special Marketing Representative: Robin Barry

ASQ Mission: The American Society for Quality advances individual, organizational, and community excellence worldwide through learning, quality improvement, and knowledge exchange.

Attention Bookstores, Wholesalers, Schools and Corporations: ASQ Quality Press books, videotapes, audiotapes, and software are available at quantity discounts with bulk purchases for business, educational, or instructional use. For information, please contact ASQ Quality Press at 800-248-1946, or write to ASQ Quality Press, P.O. Box 3005, Milwaukee, WI 53201-3005.

To place orders or to request a free copy of the ASQ Quality Press Publications Catalog, including ASQ membership information, call 800-248-1946. Visit our Web site at www.asq.org or http://qualitypress.asq.org.

 Printed on acid-free paper

Quality Press
600 N. Plankinton Avenue
Milwaukee, Wisconsin 53203
Call toll free 800-248-1946
Fax 414-272-1734
www.asq.org
http://qualitypress.asq.org
http://standardsgroup.asq.org
E-mail: authors@asq.org

ASQ
AMERICAN SOCIETY
FOR QUALITY™

This book is dedicated to Karen M. Brink for her contributions, time, and energy in assisting me in completing this project. Her tireless efforts of reviewing, critiquing, and making this book useful are deeply appreciated.

Table of Contents

List of Figures . . . . *ix*

Foreword . . . . *xi*

Introduction . . . . *xv*

**Chapter 1   Eight Keys to Creating a Sustainable Quality
Management System** **1**

The Process Model for Continual Improvement 2
The Eight Keys 2
Summary 10

**Chapter 2   Background and Introduction to the ISO 9001:2000 Family
of Standards** **13**

Introduction to ISO 9001:2000 13
ISO 9000 Series (ISO 9000, ISO 9001, and ISO 9004) 14
Restructuring and Consolidation of the ISO 9000 Family
    of Standards 14
ISO 9000:2000 15
ISO 9001:2000 and ISO 9004:2000 15
ISO 9001:2000: Clauses 0–3 16

Chapter 3   ISO 9001:2000 Clause 4—Quality Management System **21**

4.1 General Requirements 22
4.2 Documentation Requirements 23
Quality Policy, Goals and Objectives 25
4.2.1(b) and 4.2.2: The Quality Manual 25
Quality System Level Procedures and Documentation 33
Rules for Writing Procedures 35
The Quality Plan 37
Writing How-To Documents: Work Instructions and Protocols 38
4.2.1(e) Records Required 38

4.2.3 Control of Documents   38
Forms Control   40
Control of Documents of External Origin   40
4.2.4 Control of Records   41

Chapter 4   ISO 9001:2000 Clause 5—Management Responsibility **43**
5.1 Management Commitment   43
5.2 Customer Focus   43
Customer Focus—Who Is the Customer?   44
5.3 Quality Policy   45
5.4 Planning   45
5.4.1 Quality Objectives   47
5.4.2 Quality Management System Planning   48
5.5 Responsibility, Authority and Communication,
     5.5.1 Responsibility and Authority   49
5.5.2 Management Representative   49
5.5.3 Internal Communication   49
5.6 Management Review   50
5.6.2 Review Input   50
5.6.3 Review Output   51
Records of Management Review   52

Chapter 5   ISO 9001:2000 Clause 6—Resource Management **53**
6.1 Provision of Resources   53
6.2 Human Resources   53
6.3 Infrastructure and 6.4 Work Environment   54

Chapter 6   ISO 9001:2000 Clause 7—Product Realization **57**
7.1 Planning of Product Realization   57
7.2 Customer-Related Processes   58
7.2.2 Review of Requirements Related to the Product   59
7.2.3 Customer Communication   62
7.3 Design and Development   62
7.4 Purchasing, 7.4.1 Purchasing Process   64
7.4.2 Purchasing Information   66
7.4.3 Verification of Purchased Product   66
7.5 Production and Service Provision   66
7.5.2 Validation of Processes   70
7.5.3 Identification and Traceability   70
7.5.4 Customer Property   70
7.5.5 Preservation of Product   71
7.6 Control of Monitoring and Measuring Devices   72

**Chapter 7   ISO 9001:2000 Clause 8—Measurement, Analysis
and Improvement** **75**
8.1 General   75

8.2.1 Customer Satisfaction   75
8.2.2 Internal Audit   76
8.2.3 and 8.2.4 Monitoring and Measurement of Processes
    and Product   80
8.3 Control of Nonconforming Product   81
8.4 Analysis of Data   82
8.5.1 Continual Improvement   83
8.5.2 Corrective Action   83
8.5.3 Preventive Action   84

Chapter 8   Conclusion **85**
Putting All the Pieces Together   85

Appendix A   ISO 9001:2000 Self-Assessment Tool **87**
Scoring the Self-Assessment Instrument   87

Appendix B   Sample Quality Systems Manual and Procedures **107**

Appendix C   Sample Flowcharts and Process Maps **163**

References *177*

About the Author *179*

Index *181*

List of Figures

Figure 1.1   Continual improvement of the quality management system.   2

Figure 1.2   Process defined: The transformation of inputs into outputs.   7

Figure 3.1   Sequence and interaction of a healthcare process.   27

Figure 3.2   Typical hospital sequence and interaction of healthcare processes.   28

Figure 6.1   Basic flowcharting.   69

Figure 7.1   Five keys to continual improvement.   83

Foreword

If you are reading this, you have undoubtedly been in the healthcare field for some time. You may be looking at ISO 9001:2000 as just another trend in quality management. Another program your organization must explore and add to your list of quality designations. Another cost that keeps your organization competitive. However, you may also question whether you can really afford it with reimbursements dropping and hospitals merging and closing daily.

Let me assure you—an ISO 9001:2000 quality management system is not a tool to add to your list of daunting requirements. Rather, it can be the answer to the business critics who do not believe healthcare professionals can bring industry costs under control and provide Americans with the type of service they expect. It can be the answer to restoring creativity to the healthcare professionals we love and respect because of their brilliance and innovation in diagnosis and treatment. It can allow us, together, to create the new healthcare.

Healthcare is a service industry. We provide a wonderful product that heals body, mind, and soul. Almost everyone needs it at some time in their lives. Accessible, local healthcare is an integral part of the communities in which we live.

The value of preserving our health is above question.

America covets its quality healthcare. Society is asking for reassurance that that quality care will be there when control of their livelihood falls into our capable hands. Managed care has taught us much, but is not the answer. We are reminded that medicine is about people and these people are unique and complex. Healthcare is a beautiful blend of art and science. Application of across-the-board cuts, absolute rules for service, and limits on inventory do not get us where we want to be. It's just not that simple . . . and that is the challenge. So, how do we learn from the past and build trust in the future?

The missing link to all improvement efforts is accountability—individual, corporate, and community. Health professionals are taught to work independently and act with authority in making decisions. Otherwise, how could patients trust us in their time of need? That same autonomy limits our quality. This is not a criticism, just a fact. We need to develop what all the business texts call synergy: the action of two or more to achieve an effect of which each is individually incapable.

Quality can only develop to its maximum potential if we work together, become accountable to one another and our patients. We must care about how we perform our procedures in relation to the organization and others. Caregiving can lead to overcare. There is a delicate balance needed which many have failed to achieve.

So, how can ISO 9001:2000 make a real difference? It is the vehicle that can move healthcare to balance cost and quality in a positive way. It gives health professionals a common structure within which to grow toward individual and team accountability. Everyone is involved in creating a custom system for your organization. Physicians, administrators, managers, and staff are assured of a tracking mechanism for the numerous concerns that just never seem to get fixed. There is constant vigilance until satisfaction is reached because the overreaching goal of ISO 9001:2000 is customer satisfaction for all stakeholders.

Achieving this goal is only possible through committed application. ISO 9001:2000 standards must be integrated into daily work and utilized because they provide management with information crucial to assessing and solving problems effectively. Their value is in the implementation carried out by each individual. The resulting benefits increase proportionate to the level of commitment and implementation of each person involved.

To facilitate this team culture and its synergy, ISO 9001:2000 focuses on *process*. Pulling people together to map what is really happening opens the door to brainstorming. You think you understand what's going on until you sit down with your colleagues and really listen to them. How can we possibly impose successful standardization without looking at the actual process first? And, the more disciplines involved, the more innovation is possible. Creativity is unleashed and healthcare workers are allowed to influence their own environment. This, in turn, gives relief from frustration and restores hope in the organization.

Increased understanding, physician and staff buy-in, customer focus, reduced costs, joint satisfaction, healing—when it all comes together, healthcare returns to its original mission in an energizing way! The focus is on what we *can* do, instead of what we are not allowed to do. Caregivers are freed to do what they do best—fix things for better patient care! And, who better to know what is best?

The required ISO 9001:2000 internal audit system starts the dialogue between departments, breaking down those old, familiar walls that divide and cause conflict. Auditors, composed of many levels of staff, are formally trained, then assigned only to analyze departmental processes other than their own. The resulting increase in organizational knowledge is phenomenal. It allows an objective peer review and innately develops a system perspective. Understanding brings appreciation that builds teamwork to grow synergy. And it is a natural result of the ISO 9001:2000 system.

This cultural change, possible with the ISO 9001:2000 management system, is a major benefit to your organization. Just imagine how having twenty-plus quality ambassadors working throughout your organization could make a difference in a short period of time. Our dedicated, experienced associates believe in ISO 9001:2000. Our new associates are very impressed with this "cutting edge" approach (think about recruitment). Furthermore, our organization has been vitalized in a time when fear, insecurity, and overwhelming hours of work decrease morale and dominate healthcare reports in the news. Our image needs a facelift.

Is ISO 9001:2000 a fit for your organization? Like any system or structure, its success depends on you. Management commitment—*real* commitment—is needed to mobilize this system. I am convinced that ISO 9001:2000 offers an answer to the healthcare dilemma of today like nothing else that exists. It offers a unique method that can restore confidence in our business acumen and rebuild trust in the service of healing. It all depends on our resolve and commitment to believe it, apply it, and stay the course. It will take time to realize the benefits of cost control and customer satisfaction. I hope you will join us in this worthwhile endeavor. Together, we can shape the new healthcare.

Jean Smith RN, BBL, MBA
Former Vice President Operations of an
ISO 9001:2000 Certified Hospital

Introduction

It is no secret that United States healthcare organizations find themselves in difficult times. These circumstances include government cutbacks in Medicare; the rising cost of malpractice insurance; enhanced, new, and ever-changing regulations that erode organizational creativity; difficulty in attracting and keeping qualified professionals; overworked staff; enforcement and compliance requirements that tend to choke organizational effectiveness; and accreditation requirements that constantly change. The list can go on and on.

It is for these reasons that implementing an effective and efficient ISO 9001:2000 quality management system is not only advisable but also necessary. Such a management system can increase operational efficiency and enhance financial effectiveness. In addition, newly educated healthcare professionals and experienced, highly motivated people want to work in an environment that is progressive and willing to try new initiatives. They seek out organizations that have adopted a fresh approach to healthcare service delivery processes.

This introduction is not about convincing the reader to implement ISO 9001:2000. It is about explaining why the American healthcare system needs such a methodology of process management, and assisting and providing guidance to those that have decided to implement such a system. For too many years, healthcare organizations, regulators, and state hospital associations have been content with the status quo. It is time to implement a new paradigm of quality management that will bring about clear, concise, and measurable improvements; reduce medical errors and mistakes; and change the face of healthcare delivery systems.

While traveling frequently throughout the United States speaking at hundreds of hospitals, trade associations, and other types of healthcare organizations about the virtues of ISO 9001:2000 quality management systems, I am always asked the question, "How much money will I save if my organization implements an ISO 9001:2000 process management quality system?" It is strange that while preaching the ISO 9001:2000 gospel to healthcare organizations, *no* administrators have ever asked me the question, "How many lives could be saved if my organization implements an ISO 9001:2000 process-based quality management system?"

Let's look at healthcare's recent history regarding healthcare delivery processes and patient safety in light of sticking with the status quo.

In 1964, 20 percent of patients suffered an iatrogenic injury.[1] It is interesting to note that 20 percent of those injuries were either serious or fatal (Schimmel, 64). Less than 20 years later, 36 percent of patients suffered an iatrogenic injury, with 25 percent of those being serious or life threatening (Steel, 1981). In 1989, patients in medical intensive care units experienced about 1.7 errors each day (Gopher, 1989).

In 1991, one out of every 25 patients hospitalized were injured by medical errors (Brenan, 1991). Iatrogenic injuries occurred in 3.7 percent of hospitalizations. However, 70 percent were preventable (Harvard Medical Practice Study, 1991), as were 64 percent of cardiac arrests (Bedell, 1991). Medication errors caused one of every five injuries or deaths (Leape, 1991).

By 1999, surgical adverse events occurred in one of 50 admissions, accounted for two of three adverse events, and accounted for one of every eight hospital deaths (Gawande, 1999). Over time, autopsies consistently showed a 10 percent rate of diagnostic error (Bardage, 1999).

In 1984, much public attention was drawn to the Libby Zion case, in which, for the first time, prosecutors sought to bring criminal charges against physicians. The grand jury declined to return an indictment citing that there had been *system problems* within the hospital and not errors or malpractice caused by the physicians.

Several years ago, the Institute of Medicine (IOM) issued a report entitled *To Err is Human*. This report gained national press when it stated that 98,000 deaths per year were caused by medical errors. The report stated that more people die from medical error than breast cancer, HIV, or motor vehicle accidents.

What does this really mean? Doesn't this equate to an error rate that is only one percent? That seems good but let's look closer.

In manufacturing, many organizations have implemented Six Sigma methodologies that state that there are 3.4 defects (something not meeting customer requirements) per million opportunities, which is near perfect. Using the IOM report, the American healthcare system would rate a 2.8 process sigma over the short term and 1.8 over the long term. A 2.8 sigma is more than 200,000 wrong drug prescriptions per year compared to six sigma of 68 wrong prescriptions per year. A 2.8 sigma means more than 5,000 incorrect surgical procedures each week compared to six sigma of 1.7 incorrect procedures per week. So, yes, an error rate of one percent is bad.

Why all this discussion about errors and system problems? What does this have to do with implementing ISO 9001:2000? Simply put, everything. The whole purpose of the healthcare delivery system is to attempt to help sick people get well. If the processes and systems that deliver this service are not functioning properly, then the result can be tragic.

Now back to the question, "How much money will I save if the organization implements an ISO 9001:2000 process management system?"

In response, I pose a related question. How much do medical errors cost? Adverse drug events would cost $4,700 each, or $1,400,000 per year at a 350 bed hospital (Bates, 1997). Medical error costs about $5 million per year in large teaching hospitals

(Bates, 1997). Nationwide, medical errors cost about $29 billion per year (IOM, 1999). The most alarming statistic is that the cost of adverse events is similar to the national cost of caring for people with HIV/AIDS (Thomas, 1999).

If implementing an ISO 9001:2000 quality management system helps reduce medical errors, these figures represent money saved! The problem is that *prevention does not produce clear statistics!*

How can lives be saved and costs reduced? Implement an ISO 9001:2000 process approach quality management system. The IOM, as does ISO 9001:2000, cites four themes that a healthcare organization can implement to answer this question: new vision, redesigning of healthcare delivery systems, building organizational supports for change, and environmental change.

How can an organization accomplish these implementation themes? Apply ISO 9001:2000!

This book was developed to assist administrative personnel, management, quality professionals, risk managers, compliance officers, and other clinical and nonclinical staff to understand the fundamentals of implementing a sustainable management system. This system would produce a new millennium healthcare organization, increase revenues, and protect patients. An ISO 9001:2000 management system drives process management methodologies that revolve around IOM's four themes.

The book's interpretive guidance to ISO 9001:2000 in a health services context is based on the hands-on experience of the author, who, with other staff from Quality Paradigms Training & Consulting, has been consulting, implementing, and assessing healthcare organizations since ISO 9000's introduction into the healthcare sector in 1995. This book is intended for all healthcare organizations including hospitals, health systems, community-based health services, occupational health clinics, physician practices, management service organizations, medical groups, laboratories, blood banks, and clinical research organizations.

This book can also apply to specialized divisions such as training, imaging, and sterilization and to support services such as cleaning, maintenance of buildings and equipment, administration, linen services, and food and other hotel services, all of which can have a significant impact on patient care and outcomes. It must be used in conjunction with the ISO 9001:2000 standard. Additionally, the ISO International Working Agreement (IWA 1, *Guidelines for process improvements in health service organizations*) may be useful when implementing the standard. The basis for the ISO IWA 1 document is the ISO 9004:2000 document, and the ISO 9004 document should not be used for implementation or future registration. The IWA 1 document should only be used as a guideline.

This book is not intended to provide guidance on performance or outcome standards. The ISO 9001:2000 standard takes a systems and process approach to improving performance (organizational and financial) by providing a focus on quality management, process control, and quality assurance techniques to achieve planned outcomes and prevent unsatisfactory performance or nonconformance.

The examples in this book should not be taken as prescriptive or exhaustive or as preferred implementation methodology. There are many ways of achieving the intent of the ISO 9001:2000 standard, and the healthcare organization should adopt those approaches that best suit its mode of operation. Each healthcare organization should verify that the approaches it chooses to implement provide for an effective quality management system. Each healthcare organization should identify its key processes by building on existing policies, guidelines, and management control systems to develop a quality management system that is suitable for, and is structured to reflect, the scope of services it supplies and the processes and specific practices it employs.

ENDNOTE

1. Research statistics cited by the VHA in a speech to the Michigan Hospital Association Insurance Company Risk Manager's conference, August 23, 2001.

1

Eight Keys to Creating a Sustainable Quality Management System

These eight keys were developed for use by management in order to lead organizations to improved performance.

Healthcare professionals are besieged by competing requirements, heavy workloads that require more time than is available, customer concerns from various levels and for differing reasons, and business concerns that are not always within their expertise. Various driving forces from external sources surround the healthcare organization: regulators, patient/customer needs, expectations and mandates for safety, and patient/customer satisfaction. Personnel within the healthcare provider's organization attempt to drive performance and process improvement within the operation based on feedback from external sources but seldom have the time or infrastructure to do so effectively.

What is the answer for healthcare? Various healthcare initiatives have come and gone over the years, none with lasting success. In contrast, ISO 9001 certification has proven to initiate and sustain lasting change and quality improvement in a wide spectrum of industries. A robust ISO 9001:2000 quality management system is the answer for healthcare organizations.

ISO 9001:2000 is an excellent business management modeling tool that places an emphasis on managing systems, managing processes, and controlling protocols and instructions. ISO 9001:2000 can be the process management tool that busy healthcare professionals use to address the infrastructure and time issues that face them. ISO 9001:2000 provides a framework and methodology for monitoring and measuring conformity and, unlike the Malcom Baldrige National Quality Award, does not require the healthcare organization to focus energy and resources on winning an award but on defining, documenting, and implementing processes; identifying opportunities for continual improvement;

1

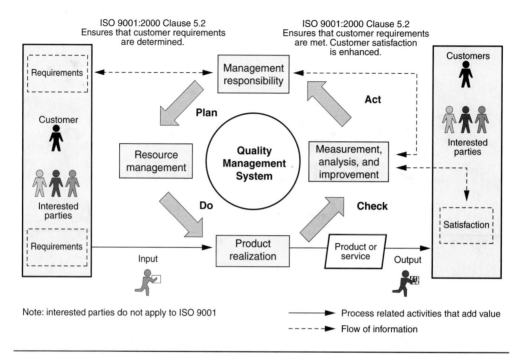

Figure 1.1   Continual improvement of the quality management system. Adapted fom ANSI/ISO/ASQ Q9001-2000, Figure 1. Used with permission.

and enhancing customer satisfaction. Implementing and maintaining a sustainable quality management system becomes the way that the organization operates. Due to the ongoing yearly assessment by a third-party certification body, the documented ISO 9001:2000 management system remains intact, viable, and always improving.

THE PROCESS MODEL FOR CONTINUAL IMPROVEMENT

The quality management system structure of ISO 9001:2000 is shown in Figure 1.1. This process management model stresses the importance of identifying patient/customer needs and expectations prior to carrying out service delivery and then delivering the agreed upon services or products. This process model also demonstrates that healthcare organizations must identify, provide, and maintain adequate resources, processes, and measures to effectively deliver the agreed upon service so that planned healthcare outcomes are achieved.

THE EIGHT KEYS

The ISO 9001:2000 standard is based on eight quality management principles. These principles become the *eight keys to improvement* for the healthcare organization. In operating any organization, it is necessary for leadership to direct, control, manage, and oversee the organization in a planned and systematic manner. Successful organizations have found that when implementing an ISO 9001:2000 quality management system, organizational performance is enhanced, and processes and practices are continually improved by truly identifying and addressing the needs of its patients/customers.

The eight keys, known as *principles,* can be used by leaders to drive the organization toward continual improvement of its processes, practices, and methodologies. These eight keys are *customer focus, leadership, involvement of people, process approach, system approach to management, continual improvement, factual approach to decision making,* and *mutually beneficial supplier relationships.*

The eight keys are the very heart and soul, the lifeblood, the foundation of an effective ISO 9001:2000 quality management system. Removing any one of these key pillars from the management system structure would cause the quality management system to weaken and eventually fail.

Key 1—Customer Focus: Be a Customer-Focused Organization

Since healthcare organizations depend on their patients/customers, their every need, both present and future, should be understood and met. The organization should strive not just to meet but also to exceed patient/customer expectations. A customer-focused organization does not place blame for problems on the patients/customers that it serves but rather identifies their needs and expectations in a proactive manner and then tries to exceed those needs and expectations through excellent service delivery. The customer/patient should be the number one priority in any organization. A sign seen in some businesses reads:

> Three Rules for a Successful Business:
> Rule 1—Take Care of the Customer
> Rule 2—Take Care of the Customer
> Rule 3—Take Care of the Customer

Every organization should take these three rules to heart. When these rules are implemented and become the way of thinking that permeates an organization, everything else seems to fit into place.

How can a healthcare organization focus on the customer when many times it is unclear just who the customer really is? In many healthcare organizations, clerical and clinical staff, administrators, and other healthcare professionals debate who the customer really is. Healthy discussion surrounds this question, not because healthcare service deliverers are confused, but because of the complex and multifaceted nature of the healthcare organization and its organizational components and infrastructure.

Boards of directors focus on the community at large as the healthcare organization's primary customer. Hospital administrators many times identify the physician as the primary customer due to the fact that the physician brings patients to the hospital. Clinical and support staff identify the patient as the primary customer since that is the population that they serve. Social workers and clergy focus on patients and their family members' physical, emotional, and spiritual needs. Billing personnel focus on payers and insurance companies as their primary customers. Risk managers and quality managers focus on collecting, collating, and reporting organizational improvement data, clinical outcomes, and other related data to accreditation and regulatory bodies and to the organization's administration and board of directors. The list goes on and on, and so does the debate.

When implementing an ISO 9001:2000 quality management system, one of the first tasks is to understand and identify who a healthcare organization's customers are so that customer awareness can be communicated to all employees. ISO 9000 defines the customer as an organization or person that receives the service; for example, a consumer, client, or end user. The customer can be either internal or external to the healthcare organization.

ANSI/ISO/ASQ Q9001-2000 Clause 5.2, entitled Customer focus, requires that top management, "ensure that customer requirements are determined and are met with the aim of enhancing *customer satisfaction*."[1]* How can any organization truly meet this ISO 9001:2000 requirement if it has not first identified its customers? It is vitally important to ensure that customers are identified so that the healthcare organization can enhance satisfaction. The identification of customers is the first key to implementing a sustainable quality management system in any healthcare organization. Administration must come together with staff to clearly and unambiguously identify in writing the organization's customer base whether that base is internal or external. If the identified customer base is too narrow, then the organization will not serve all of its patients/customers and other interested parties to the fullest. Because all people within the organization are essential to carrying out the organization's mission and vision, then all customers must be identified with the aim of enhancing satisfaction.

Key 2—Leadership: Provide Effective Leadership

The key role for leadership within the healthcare organization must be to establish unity of purpose, direction, and a good working environment within the organization. Leadership must create an environment in which all staff and employees can become fully involved in achieving the healthcare organization's goals, strategies, and objectives. The old saying, "Everything rises and falls on leadership" could not be truer. The traditional leadership methodology of controlling and prescribing how work will be accomplished, commanding and telling employees what to do, expecting obedience, judging and sizing up employees' performance by doling out rewards and punishments, and guarding turf while hoarding resources is still alive and well throughout America's healthcare organizations. Dwight D. Eisenhower once said, "You do not lead by hitting people over the head—that's assault, not leadership." Such leadership tactics cause organizations to become dysfunctional. New methods *must* be nurtured.

The new high-involvement leadership paradigm is very slow at gaining understanding by healthcare administrators and managers. As high-involvement leadership

---

* ANSI/ISO/ASQ Q9001-2000 is a verbatim adoption for the U.S. market of the ISO 9001:2000 standard.

takes hold, these dysfunctional methods will become obsolete. Roles that facilitate high-involvement leadership must take hold. There are several ways to facilitate high-involvement leadership within the healthcare organization.

Discover New Ways

Leadership must enforce the *one best way* of working whenever possible. As work processes are identified, defined, and documented, it is important to know where flexibility and creative problem solving are not only possible but demanded. The required work process steps must, by their very definition, be adhered to at all times. ISO 9001:2000 requires each organization to determine the sequence and interactions of its processes in order to facilitate change and bring about improvement. By utilizing the one best way philosophy, variation in work flow, work practices, and processes will be reduced, thereby causing errors to be reduced. Leaders must encourage and empower direct reports and other personnel to bring forth the best work and process practice ideas. Leaders must also seek new and better ways of accomplishing the mission; leaders must be visionary.

Make the Path Clear

In contrast to traditional leaders, the high-involvement leader must illuminate and light the path where the organization should be headed. Notice that this type of leader lights up the path but does not use a spotlight in order to see miles ahead. The focus is on the path and not the final destination. The leader must understand what the final destination is but lead the organization to that destination in small manageable increments, illuminating the path so others may follow. The leader leads the organization in small steps with the knowledge and vision of what lies ahead in the darkness.

Encourage Others along the Way

Implementing ISO 9001:2000 requires the leader to assume some degree of risk. This added risk requires employees also to assume risk and added responsibility. The high-involvement leader needs to be vocal in support of the ISO 9001:2000 initiative and not only talk about the process but become actively involved and visible throughout the implementation project. Encouragement is needed to keep the ISO 9001:2000 implementation project on track and to ensure that people understand the importance of implementing a sustainable quality management system. On the Web site www.motivational-inspirational-corner.com/getquote.html?catagoryid=114, Jim Stovall sums it up this way: "You need to be aware of what others are doing, applaud their efforts, acknowledge their successes, and encourage them in their pursuits. When we all help one another, everybody wins."

Key 3—Involvement of People: Many People Must Be Involved

Since organizations are comprised of people, a healthcare organization achieves maximum benefit when its employees are fully involved and using their abilities to the organization's advantage.

As leadership lilluminates the pathway to where the organization is headed, people will better understand the importance of their role within the organization. This often happens only after people begin to see how implementation of an ISO 9001:2000 quality management system can create a positive effect and impact the jobs and duties that they carry out day-to-day. An effectively implemented ISO 9001:2000 quality management system should make people's jobs easier to perform and less redundant. At this point, people typically become more intimately involved in identifying methods for improving the processes they own. As leadership creates an environment where employees are allowed to become more involved in the decision making process, personnel naturally become more highly motivated and committed to the organization. Greater employee involvement results in greater innovation and creativity that furthers the organization's goals, strategies, and objectives. People tend to become more accountable for their own performance and are eager to participate in and contribute to continual improvement. The greater the involvement, the more successful an organization will be.

Key 4—The Process Approach: Identify and Manage the Process

The healthcare organization's primary desire is to achieve greater efficiency when organizational resources and work practices, protocols, and activities are managed as a process. Figure 1.1 illustrates the ISO 9001:2000 process management model. A process is the steps and actions necessary for transforming inputs into outputs. The output from one process often forms the input for another.

Let's look at one example: a patient is discharged from surgery and admitted to the nursing unit. The patient's chart (the process input document) is delivered to the nursing unit. The nursing unit provides the required care to the patient (the care delivery process). The patient is provided postsurgery education and subsequently discharged (the process output—process completed).

The medical chart (the coding process input document) is forwarded to the coding department. The coding department completes coding and the medical chart (the coding process output—process completed) is forwarded to the medical records department.

The medical records department receives the medical chart (medical records process input), checks, logs, records (processes), and files the record (medical records process output—process complete). See Figure 1.2.

Leadership must develop a process approach to managing the healthcare organization's processes and internal management system infrastructure. Processes need to be defined and documented in order to better understand the linkage between process and the work flow and the interactions that take place at the handoffs between corresponding processes. Once process work flow is understood, improvements can be made when variation in process work flow is identified and change is found necessary. Understanding and documenting the process flow of work also provides new employees with the opportunity to learn their jobs more quickly, thereby limiting the number of errors made. As discussed earlier, using the one best way philosophy, along with

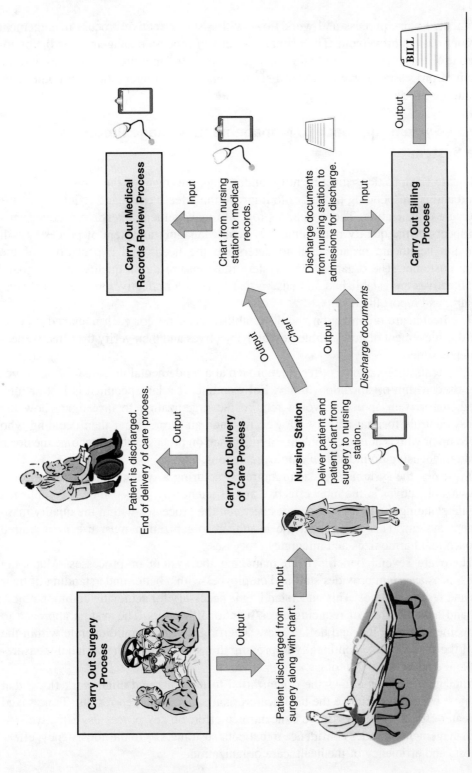

Figure 1.2   Process defined: the transformation of inputs into outputs.

documented work process and work flow, will ensure effective process management and continual improvement. The primary benefit of process management is the ongoing control that it provides over the linkage between the individual processes and the system of processes, as well as over their combination and interaction with other corresponding processes.

Key 5—System Approach to Management: Manage Processes As a System

Healthcare organizations must identify, understand, and manage their system of interrelated and corresponding processes to improve the effectiveness and efficiency of the healthcare organization. The system approach to management takes into account various aspects of the quality management system. Managing a system of processes will cause the healthcare organization to determine the needs and expectations of the patient/customer. The organization's system must ensure that a quality policy, goals, and objectives are established and ensure that there is an effective process to achieve, measure, and report the results.

The healthcare organization should establish measures for each managed process toward achievement of goals, strategies, and objectives and then verify the effectiveness of the measures.

A systems approach is a different approach at a fundamental level than what is typically used within organizations today. For example, if a lab specimen is lost or misplaced, the system approach would require the organization to investigate how the process controls for that activity allowed for such an error, rather than deciding who slipped up or who is at fault. Problem solving based on process should become the norm instead of focusing on individual employee actions.

Typically, the systems approach requires structuring a system to achieve the organization's objectives in the most effective and efficient way. This can be accomplished by understanding the interdependencies between the processes within the quality management system. This means that the healthcare organization must use a structured approach that harmonizes and integrates processes.

There are several benefits from managing the system of processes. Managing processes as a system provides staff and employees with a better understanding of their roles and responsibilities. This understanding is necessary for achieving common objectives and has the effect of reducing cross-functional barriers. The system approach to management also targets and defines how specific activities should operate within the rest of the system while continually improving that system through continual measurement and evaluation of outcomes.

Managing systems allows the organization to integrate and align work flows that will most efficiently achieve the healthcare organization's desired results. Time saved by greater efficiency allows more concentrated effort on key processes. Effective system management provides confidence to patients/customers as to the consistency, effectiveness, and efficiency of the healthcare organization.

Key 6—Continual Improvement: It Can Always Be Improved

Continual improvement should be the permanent objective of every healthcare provider. Every activity that is repeated can be improved. A suggestion for improvement is not a statement of failure in the past but of improvement for the future.

The problem with improvement is that while it is undeniably a good idea, human emotions interfere with intellect when the suggestion is made that there may be a better way to do things. The present method was someone's good idea in the past. That person may still be in charge of the process under discussion and may feel like someone is finding fault with his or her work. The culture for improvement is not automatic. It is achieved over time by educating employees at every opportunity that excellence can be improved upon and that a suggestion for improvement is not by nature a criticism of what was done in the past.

Key 7—Factual Approach to Decision Making: Decisions Are Made Based on Data

The healthcare organization must base decisions on logical or intuitive data that has been analyzed. Here is a case in point: If specific data is not gathered on dispensing medication, there is no way to know the impact of a deviation. Suppose a medication error occurs. As a result of this one occurrence, the physician responsible for the patient in question may feel that the entire hospital is fraught with errors. This physician then creates a community- and/or hospitalwide backlash suggesting the nursing staff is incompetent and uncaring. The nursing staff knows that the situation in question never put the patient in danger and that the error was not a recurring problem but was extremely unusual.

In this fictitious case, the nursing staff could not prove or demonstrate that a prior error had not occurred nor did they have evidence of their normally excellent record in dispensing medications. The hospital, in response to the physician's statements and community concern, launched a time-consuming and expensive study on the nursing staff's qualifications and training in medication protocols.

In contrast, a data-driven system would be capable of analyzing the impact and frequency. (Was a common pain reliever delivered at the wrong time or a potentially life-threatening substance given in error?)

While the goal must obviously be zero errors, real-time data creates a realistic and true perspective instead of an emotional response. In the sample case, hospital administration took action to correct a problem that may not have been an ongoing concern. If the emphasis had been to investigate and identify methods to collect data and then determine appropriate corrective action, the response may have been more appropriate.

Most healthcare providers do not suffer from a lack of data. Instead, there is often an abundance of data, but a failure to use the data for a practical purpose. It is important to have a purpose for data. If staff members required to collect data perceive their effort as a waste of time, they may not be accurate, may not be timely in reporting, and may eventually cease data collection altogether.

Key 8—Mutually Beneficial Supplier Relationships: Create Working Relationships with Suppliers

Relationships between the healthcare organization and their suppliers must be structured to benefit both parties in order to enhance the ability of the healthcare organization and its suppliers to create value for customers. Suppliers for healthcare organizations are often sole sources or large purchasing contractors whose organizations choose multiple vendors to get the best price for the healthcare organization. These healthcare organization/supplier relationships must be structured to benefit the healthcare provider instead of holding the purchasing system captive to arrangements that no longer serve the original purpose. How are supplier complaints communicated? Do suppliers respond? Does the resolution provide benefit for both parties?

The problem with supplier relationships is that many such arrangements are independent of the established purchasing process. Many managers have private arrangements with subcontractors, they may use credit cards for small purchases, or managers may feel that each case is special and falls outside of the normal guidelines. Managers are often skilled at circumventing the system. As a result, it can be very difficult to control spending and, ultimately, difficult to determine profitability in the best case; in the worst case, the purchase of inferior supplies and equipment or contracts with unsuitable or unqualified providers may impact the quality of service.

SUMMARY

The ISO 9001:2000 standard organizes eight keys, known as management principles, into five main clauses of requirements. The requirements for implementing an ISO 9001:2000 quality management system are located in Clauses 4–8 (five clauses and subclauses).

When a healthcare organization is audited for compliance to the ISO 9001:2000 standard, implementation of all quality management system clauses must be evaluated. The five main quality management system requirements are as follows:

- Clause 4—Quality management system

- Clause 5—Management responsibility (leadership)

- Clause 6—Resource management (people, facilities, equipment)

- Clause 7—Product realization (process identification and process management)

- Clause 8—Measurement, analysis and improvement (improvement for patient/customer satisfaction)

These five main clauses describe the quality management system requirements that the healthcare organizations must implement in order to achieve ISO 9001:2000 compliance. These five clauses will be discussed in the following chapters.

The process management philosophy of the ISO 9001:2000 standard (see Figure 1.1) begins with its focus on customer/patient requirements: everything to do with quality starts and ends with the customer/patient. What the customer/patient wants, needs, and expects becomes a basis for the input into the quality management system. This input feeds into the service planning process and finally into requirements for service delivery. Management responsibility (leadership), resource management (people, facilities, and equipment), product realization (process), and measurement, analysis and improvement (improvement for customer/patient satisfaction) describe the requirements that organizations must implement in order to deliver quality services using a systematic standard approach.

The actual delivery of healthcare service becomes the organization's process output. The healthcare organization is then required to evaluate pertinent information on customer/patient perception and satisfaction (or dissatisfaction). This can be accomplished by implementing Clause 8—Measurement, analysis and improvement. Measurements and evaluations become feedback on a healthcare organization's ability to meet customer/patient requirements. The healthcare organization is required to measure and monitor both service delivery processes and the service delivery itself. Satisfaction measures are used as feedback to evaluate and validate whether customer/patient requirements have been met.

The ISO 9001:2000 quality management system is comprised of quality policy, quality objectives, procedure documents, policies, and records. The quality management system is the documented infrastructure, the heart of the management system. All processes and activities revolve around the documented quality management system.

ENDNOTES

1. Customer satisfaction is the customer's perception of the degree to which the customer's requirements have been fulfilled. Customer complaints are an indicator of low customer satisfaction but their absence does not necessarily imply high customer satisfaction. Even when all of the customer's requirements have been agreed to and fulfilled, it does not assure high customer satisfaction.

2

Background and Introduction to the ISO 9001:2000 Family of Standards

Organizational processes remain static until they are written down to describe what happens. Only then can true change take place.

INTRODUCTION TO ISO 9001:2000

What is ISO? ISO is derived from the Greek word *isos* meaning *all sides are equal.* ISO documents were drafted by the International Organization for Standardization to ensure the uniformity and harmonization of standards that had proliferated around the world. The ISO 9000 series (ISO 9000:2000, ISO 9001:2000, and ISO 9004:2000) are quality management system standards that define minimum requirements and can be applied to any and all organizations.

The ISO 9000 series of standards has quickly become the international language of quality. Since its first issue in 1987, the ISO 9000 series of quality management system standards has been adopted throughout Europe, Asia, the United States, and other parts of the world as the standard for quality system certification and registration. Indeed, there is unanimous worldwide acceptance of these standards as quality management system standards.

The International Organization for Standardization is headquartered in Geneva, Switzerland, with over 120 member countries. These member countries have adopted the ISO 9000 series as their country's national standard for quality management systems. In the United States, the U.S. Department of Commerce issues national standards through the American National Standards Institute (ANSI), the ISO representative in the United States. ANSI has authorized the U.S. equivalent version of the ISO 9000 series, known as ANSI/ISO/ASQ Q9000, Q9001, and Q9004. These documents are equivalent to the international version of ISO 9000, 9001, and 9004.

ISO 9000 SERIES (ISO 9000, ISO 9001, AND ISO 9004)

The ISO 9000 series of standards were issued in 1987 and were revised for the first time in 1994. In 1997, discussion began regarding a 2000 revision to the standards. ISO technical committees investigating the revision conducted a global survey of users and registered companies of the ISO standards to better understand their needs. This survey process of 1120 companies covered attitudes towards the existing standards, requirements for the revised standards, and the relationship between the quality management system standards and the environmental management system standards.

Feedback from users and customers determined the following needs:

- The revised standards should be simple to use, easy to understand, and use clear language and terminology.

- The revised standards should have a common structure based on a process model.

- ISO 9001 requirements should include demonstration of continuous improvement and prevention of nonconformity.

- The revised standards should be suitable for all sizes of organizations, operate in any economic or industrial sector, and the manufacturing language and focus of the 1994 standards should be removed.

- Provision should be made for the exclusion of requirements that do not apply to an organization.

- The revised standards should facilitate self-evaluation and self-assessment.

- The revised standards should have increased compatibility with the ISO 14000 series of environmental management system standards.

- ISO 9001 should address effectiveness while ISO 9004 should address both efficiency and effectiveness.

- ISO 9004 should help achieve benefits for all interested parties: customers, owners, employees, suppliers and society.

To ensure that the revised standards satisfied these user and customer needs, a validation process was implemented. The validation process allowed for direct feedback from users and customers at key milestones during the revision process to determine how well these needs were being met and to identify opportunities for improvement.

RESTRUCTURING AND CONSOLIDATION OF THE ISO 9000 FAMILY OF STANDARDS

By the end of year 2000, the ISO 9000 family of standards contained more than 20 separate standards documents. This proliferation of quality system standards had been a particular concern of ISO 9000 users because the original intent in creating an international standard was to produce a single standard to be used by all. To respond to this concern, the ISO technical committee agreed that the ISO 9000 family of standards should consist of only three primary standards. The key points in the former 20 clauses of the ISO 9001 standard were to be integrated into the three primary standards, thereby allowing specific sector needs to be addressed while maintaining the universal nature of the standards. The three primary standards are:

1. ISO 9000:2000, Quality management systems—Fundamentals and vocabulary

2. ISO 9001:2000, Quality management systems—Requirements

3. ISO 9004:2000, Quality management systems—Guidelines for performance improvements

ISO 9000:2000

The former ISO 8402 quality vocabulary standard was revised to become the ISO 9000:2000 standard. This standard includes an introduction to quality management fundamentals and concepts as well as a revised vocabulary and glossary of terms.

ISO 9001:2000 AND ISO 9004:2000

The 1994 versions of ISO 9001, ISO 9002, and ISO 9003 standards are consolidated into the single revised ISO 9001 standard. The revised ISO 9001 and ISO 9004 standards were developed as a *consistent pair* of standards. The term *consistent pair* describes the structure of the documents; they are numbered consistently, so it is clear that the guidance in ISO 9004 corresponds to the ISO 9001 section with the same number. The revised ISO 9001 clearly addresses the quality management system requirements. In contrast, the revised ISO 9004 standard is intended to lead beyond the mere implementation of ISO 9001 to the development of a more comprehensive and efficient quality management system. The revised ISO 9004 is not an implementation guide for ISO 9001 implementation. It points the way to the achievement of a higher level of performance.

Tailoring of ISO 9001:2000 requirements is permitted to omit requirements that do not apply to an organization. However, any exclusions that are claimed by an organization must be thoroughly justified within the quality manual (discussed later). An exclusion is not a choice made by the organization that it will not comply with a requirement; instead, an exclusion is the identification of a requirement that cannot be complied with because the nature of the business makes it impossible to meet the requirement. For example, an organization that never handles customer property cannot apply the requirements in 7.5.4 Customer property.

The ISO 9001:2000 and ISO 9004:2000 standards have been developed using a simple process-based structure. This is a departure from the previous ISO 9001:1994

20-clause structure. This new process-based management system structure approach is consistent with Dr. Deming's plan–do–check–act improvement cycle (refer to Figure 1.1 on page 2). The major clause titles in the ISO 9001:2000 standards are:

- Clause 4—Quality management system (process management, documentation, records)

- Clause 5—Management responsibility (policy, objectives, planning, responsibility and authority, documentation, communications, and management review)

- Clause 6—Resource management (human resources, infrastructure and work environment)

- Clause 7—Product realization (customer requirements, design, purchasing, production and service operations, and calibration)

- Clause 8—Measurement, analysis and improvement (audit, satisfaction, inspection and testing, nonconformity, corrective and preventive action, and continuous improvement)

Since Figure 1.1 is a model of the complete quality management system processes, it is capable of demonstrating both vertical and horizontal process integration in a closed-loop manner.

For a vertical loop example, management defines requirements under Management responsibility. Necessary resources (physical, equipment, personnel, supplies) are determined and applied within Resource management. Processes are identified, planned, established, and implemented under Product realization. Satisfaction, performance, and improvement results are measured and analyzed, and the quality management system is thus improved through Measurement, analysis and improvement.

Management review of management system performance closes the loop, the complete cycle returns to Management responsibility for change authorization and initiation of improvement efforts.

As an example of a horizontal loop, the continual improvement model recognizes the fact that patients/customers play a significant role during the identification of needs, expectations, and requirements. Product realization processes are then carried out, and customer satisfaction is evaluated at the time of process output. This output data is then used by management to identify and improve future customer input requirements, completing the closure of the horizontal process loop.

ISO 9001:2000: CLAUSES 0–3

The ISO 9001:2000 Standard is 23 pages in length and begins with a brief foreword and an introduction (Clause 0). The foreword describes what ISO is, the technical aspects of the standards writing process, and other basic information related to the committees that created and revised the standard.

Clause 0—Introduction

The Introduction contains a description of the ISO 9001:2000 process approach, the plan–do–check–act cycle, the model of a process-based quality management system, the roles that customers play, customer satisfaction measurement, the relationship between ISO 9001:2000 and ISO 9004:2000, and a brief description of the relationship of ISO 9001:2000 and its compatibility with other management system standards.

Clause 1—Scope

As with any national or international standard, there must be a description of what activities and requirements are to be covered by the standard. The scope of ISO 9001:2000 focuses its management system requirements around two primary key purposes:

1. A quality management system should be implemented where the healthcare organization must demonstrate its ability to consistently provide healthcare-related services that meet both patient/customer and regulatory requirements.

2. A quality management system should be created where the healthcare organization's chief purpose and aim is to enhance patient/customer satisfaction through the effective implementation and application of the quality management system. This includes the healthcare organization's focus on improving processes used for continually improving its operation and assuring strict conformance to patient/customer and applicable regulatory requirements.

Clause 1 of ISO 9001:2000 provides a brief description of how the ISO standard should be applied and provides allowances for the healthcare organization to exclude specific ISO 9001:2000 requirements from the quality management system due to the nature of the services provided. If exclusions are taken, they must be justified accordingly in the quality manual.

Clause 2—Normative references

Normative references are made to other standards whose requirements constitute actual provisions of the ISO 9001:2000 standard. ISO 9000:2000 *Quality management systems— Fundamentals and vocabulary* are incorporated by reference in the standard.

Clause 3—Terms and definitions

As with all new areas of endeavor, vocabulary and concepts may need some explanation for those who find them unfamiliar. Terms and definitions for the certification standard are found in ISO 9000:2000.

Healthcare personnel often find the ISO standard confusing because some terms use familiar words that have specific meaning for quality management systems. These terms need to be defined for healthcare providers to aid in their understanding of the ISO 9001:2000 standard. Following are key terms along with their definition and some examples from healthcare settings.

Product: The Result of a Process

The standard identifies a product as one of the following:

- A service (counseling, physical therapy, nursing care and healthcare delivery)

- Hardware (oxygen tanks, wheelchairs, and so on)

- Processed materials (pharmaceutical formularies, IV solutions, blood products)

Whether the product is called a service, hardware, or processed material depends on the product being offered. For example, the offered product *automobile* consists of hardware (tires), processed materials (fuel, cooling liquid), and service (operating instructions given by the salesman).

Service delivery processes are the result of at least one activity performed at the interface between the healthcare organization and customer. Such service delivery is generally intangible. This means that the service provider and/or the patient/customer may not see the effects or outcomes of the delivered service until long after it has been delivered.

Hardware is generally tangible, and its amount is a countable characteristic (10 wheelchairs, 15 IV pumps). Processed materials are generally tangible, and their amount is also a countable characteristic (pharmaceutical formularies—medications and IV solutions). Hardware and processed materials often are referred to as goods.

Healthcare Service Delivery

Service delivery is the result of a documented or nondocumented activity generated at the interface between personnel within the healthcare organization and the patient/customer. Healthcare delivery must meet the patient/customer's holistic needs. The services provided are the result of planned activities; the healthcare organization or the patient/customer may be represented at the service delivery interface by family members, friends, healthcare personnel, or even medical equipment. The healthcare organization's service delivery interface with the patient/customer is essential to establishing an effective healthcare delivery system. Customer focus is a critical key for success.

Process

A process is a set of interrelated or interacting activities that transform inputs into outputs. Inputs into a process are generally the outputs of other processes. Processes within the healthcare organization are generally planned and carried out under controlled conditions. Such controlled conditions add value to the organization. A process or practice in which the conformity of the resulting service delivery output cannot be readily or economically verified until after service has been delivered is frequently referred to as a *special process* and must be validated to ensure consistency in the future.

System

A system is a set of interrelated or interacting elements. A healthcare system, as most healthcare providers know the term, is a single organization comprising several locations where services are provided. A healthcare system may comprise several hospitals, physician practices, and/or clinics with a single provider name. In a similar fashion, a quality management system is singular, with many functions that make up the system. The functions in a quality management system are processes; all of the processes must be managed interactively to form an effective system.

Customer

A customer is an organization or a person that receives a service. This book uses the term *patient/customer* to describe patients and other customers of a healthcare organization. The term *customer,* as used in ISO 9001:2000, can refer to any or all of the following:

- A patient
- A patient's family
- Physicians
- A surgeon, specialist, visiting medical officer, allied health professional, or other healthcare organization
- A company or organization that has contracted with the provider
- A government department
- Healthcare fund
- Another healthcare provider
- An internal customer (within the healthcare organization)
- Relevant society or community group

Customer Property

Customer property includes products that belong to a customer, patient belongings, or personal effects that are handled by the provider at any point in provision of service.

Nonconformity (Occurrence or Incident)

Nonconformity occurs with the nonfulfillment of a specified requirement. Failure to meet specified requirements may range from a physician's order not being followed to medication errors. Nonconformities (needle pricks, patient injuries, failure to administer medication, wrong medications, and so on) may be recorded on incident reports, nonconformance reports, and/or occurrence reports.

The definition of *nonconformity* also includes the absence of one or more process input/output characteristics, specified or obligatory requirements, or management system requirements; that is, an unsatisfactory outcome or failure to supply acceptable services to a patient/customer or the failure to comply with an established quality management system requirement or procedure (see ISO 9001:2000 Clause 8.3).

Review of Customer Requirements

A planned and systematic review of agreements and patient requirements (physician orders, admissions counseling, patient education service agreements, discharge counseling) that should be carried out by the healthcare organization's administration, management, or other assigned personnel prior to providing the service. These reviews should take place before signing any contract or agreement in order to ensure that all requirements for services and service delivery are adequately defined and can be met. Such reviews can be carried out jointly with the patient/customer and can be repeated at various stages during the healthcare delivery continuum. Examples of reviewing patient/customer requirements include the review of surgical services with admissions personnel, or the anesthesiologist, during patient preadmission testing. Also included are administrative review of agreements, contracts, and/or credentialing documents for anesthesiologists, doctors, and pathologists that are contracted to provide services prior to engagement.

Medical Record

Medical records are compiled by physicians and other healthcare professionals and include a patient's medical history, present illness, findings on examination, details of treatment, and notes on progress. The medical record is the legal record of care.[1]

Medical Policies and Procedures

A medical policy or procedure is any act, method, or course of action prescribed by a way of doing something, such as policies and procedures governing the medical staff credentialing process.[2]

ENDNOTES

1. Joint Commission on Accreditation of Healthcare Organizations (JCAHO) definition.
2. JCAHO definition.

3

ISO 9001:2000 Clause 4—
Quality Management System

*The system approach to management: healthcare organizations
should identify, understand, and manage a system of interrelated
processes for a given objective.*

Chapters 3 through 7 of this book will discuss each of the ISO 9001:2000 clause requirements in detail and describe how the healthcare organization should implement the requirements. Subclauses are identified by their number.

The requirements for delivering healthcare-related services must be clearly defined by the organization. Many different types of service delivery processes are involved within the daily operation of healthcare facilities. These varied delivery processes should be defined in terms of specific service characteristics or service deliverables. These deliverables or characteristics may not always be observable to the patient/customer but may affect service delivery performance outputs or create a negative impact on clinical outcomes and/or outcome measures. Healthcare service deliverables or characteristics may be quantifiable (measurable) or qualitative (comparable):

- The healthcare facility's physical plant, number of beds, and number of personnel (quantifiable)

- Waiting time, delivery time of service, and processing time (quantifiable)

- Hygiene, safety, reliability, and security (qualitative)

- Responsiveness, accessibility, courtesy, comfort, aesthetics of the environment, competence, and effective communication (qualitative)

All processes that are used to deliver services must be controlled. Good control ensures that remedial (corrective) action is possible during the actual delivery of the service. It is usually not possible to rely on the final patient assessment to influence service quality at the patient/customer interface. It is typically at this interface where customers or patients assess nonconforming conditions.

The delivery of healthcare services is highly personalized. The more definable and controlled the healthcare processes are, the greater the opportunity to apply structured and disciplined quality management system principles.

4.1 GENERAL REQUIREMENTS

The general requirements of ISO 9001:2000 are contained in Subclause 4.1. This clause sets forth all-purpose requirements relating to quality management systems and their application. It requires that the healthcare organization "establish, document, implement, and maintain" a quality management system and then continually improve that system. When establishing, documenting, and implementing a quality management system, a healthcare organization needs to establish a cross-functional team that can identify critical processes necessary for implementing an effective quality management system. As the team identifies the needed processes, they should also determine the sequence and interaction of each acknowledged process. It is vitally important for the team to ensure that all handoffs between corresponding processes are identified and documented; the majority of mistakes and errors occur at the handoffs between functions and processes.

Once the team has determined and documented the processes within the quality management system, and identified and documented the sequence and interaction of each process, the team must then determine what criteria and methods the organization will implement to ensure that the provision of healthcare services and the processes that define those services are effectively carried out.

Administration must be actively involved in the planning and implementation of the quality management system. The cross-functional team, in conjunction with the administrative team, must identify all required resources and provide any information that is deemed necessary to support the healthcare delivery system. The team should also identify which critical processes must be monitored and what resources and information are needed to implement those processes.

The cross-functional team, in conjunction with administration, risk management, and continual improvement personnel, should plan, establish, and carry out a robust internal self-assessment program. That program will be used to monitor, measure, and analyze processes within the quality management system in order to facilitate continual improvement of processes and practices within the healthcare delivery system. This internal self-assessment process is known in ISO 9001:2000 as internal auditing. The main purpose of such a self-assessment process is to ensure that the organization's defined activities, goals, policies, objectives, strategies, processes, and practices achieve planned results and that the healthcare delivery processes can be improved upon. Such a system will assist the organization in reducing variation in process performance by identifying potential and/or actual system breakdowns before critical errors and life-threatening mistakes happen.

4.2 DOCUMENTATION REQUIREMENTS

A careful review of the ANSI/ISO/ASQ Q9001-2000 standard indicates that the requirement for documenting quality management system procedures for each area is conspicuously absent. Subclause 4.2 Documentation requirements states:

The quality management system documentation shall include

    a) documented statements of a quality policy and quality objectives,

    b) a quality manual,

    c) documented procedures required by this International Standard,

    d) documents needed by the organization to ensure the effective planning, operation and control of its processes, and

    e) records required by this International Standard.

When establishing a quality management system, there are two primary types of documents that the organization must create: documented procedures required by the ISO 9001:2000 standard and documents required by the organization. The ISO 9001:2000 standard specifically requires that certain mandatory (documented) procedures be written. The following procedures are required to be established, documented, implemented, and maintained:

- 4.2.3 Control of documents
- 4.2.4 Control of records
- 8.2.2 Internal audit
- 8.3 Control of nonconforming product
- 8.5.2 Corrective action
- 8.5.3 Preventive action

These are the only subclauses within the ISO 9001:2000 standard that require a documented procedure.

The ISO 9001:2000 standard provides a healthcare organization some flexibility in establishing its quality management system documentation by indicating that these documented procedures will depend upon the particular size and type of services the organization provides, the complexity of actions and interactions of the processes being carried out, and competency of the personnel. Remember, wherever the standard refers to the words *documented procedure* it is expected that a corresponding written procedure will be provided as to how the activity or process is to be carried out.

Subclause 4.2 of the ISO 9001:2000 standard uses the term *documents* to identify how the organization will provide the information people need to perform and carry out the activities (processes) within the healthcare setting.[1] The term *documents* is intended to provide a less onerous requirement on the organization. The ISO 9001:2000 standard allows the organization to document in any form or method desired and to explain the order and interaction of the quality management system processes being used to ensure that all services offered meet patient/customer and regulatory requirements.

This does not necessarily mean that every process within the healthcare setting must be written down or covered by documents. It may be necessary for a healthcare organization to describe how some of the practices and processes are undertaken and what controls are placed on those processes in order to actually carry out critical processes. Documents can be in any form and may vary enormously from required formal healthcare accreditation documents. Documents may be photos, posters, audiotapes, video, or may be of an external nature. They may also be a model or sample documents contained on computer hard disks, diskettes, or CD-ROM. The choice is yours.

Both documented procedures (required by ISO 9001:2000) and documents (required by the healthcare organization) should indicate, to the extent necessary, who does what, where, when, why, and how. Excessive detail in procedures and other documents does not necessarily ensure more control over the process, practice, or activity. In fact, excessive detail should be avoided unless it provides value to the process, practice, or activity. Highly trained personnel with the necessary job skills to carry out a particular function or activity may reduce the need for overly detailed process control documents, provided everyone conducting the process or activity has the information needed to do the job correctly.

It is essential when implementing an effective ISO 9001:2000 quality management system within a healthcare organization to begin with the applicable ISO 9001:2000 requirements: needs or expectations that are stated, generally implied or obligatory. Most organizations begin their work by creating ISO 9001:2000 documentation *before* they really understand what is needed and end up with far more documentation than the standard requires. The ISO 9001:2000 standard requirements make reference to various plans, procedures, instructions, and the types of information described in Table 3.1.

Table 3.1 ANSI/ISO/ASQ Q9001-2000 requirements.

Clause	Required Information
4 Quality management system	Quality policy and objectives, statements, quality manual, procedures, records, and requirements
5 Management responsibility	Statutory and regulatory requirements, quality policy and objectives, requirements, plans, review inputs and outputs, customer feedback, and results
6 Resource management	Requirements, records, procedures, and results
7 Product realization	Plans, requirements, objectives, data, product information, contracts, inquiries, orders, criteria, records, work instructions, and statutory, regulatory, and other requirements
8 Measurement, analysis and improvement	Plans, procedures, results, planned arrangements, measurements, data, and requirements

All of these requirements must be recorded or documented, measured, monitored, and reviewed, but only *one* (Subclause 4.2 Documentation requirements) defines the types of documents that are required within the quality management system.

The cross-functional team should define the documentation that is deemed absolutely necessary and needed to support current processes and operations within the healthcare delivery system.

QUALITY POLICY, GOALS AND OBJECTIVES

The first set of documents that needs to be created within a healthcare organization's quality management system are the documented statements of a quality policy and quality objectives. Organizationwide goals and objectives must be identified and documented in support of the quality policy. Many healthcare organizations currently have mission and vision statements in place. These statements may be used in lieu of creating a new quality policy (see chapter 5 for additional information on the quality policy and quality objectives). For those healthcare organizations that have not established a mission or vision statement, or those that wish to create a policy statement regarding quality, a quality policy will have to be established, documented, communicated, and authorized by the administrative team. Objectives for meeting the quality policy must also be documented. When identifying and creating organizational goals and objectives, they must be SMART: specific, measurable, attainable, reasonable, and timely.

When establishing and documenting objectives, administration should consider such things as the organization's current and future business needs, products and/or services provided, organizational process performance, current satisfaction of patients/customers, and resources needed to meet the planned objectives.

4.2.1(B) AND 4.2.2: THE QUALITY MANUAL

ISO 9001:2000 Subclauses 4.2 b and 4.2.2 require that a *quality manual* be established and maintained. A quality manual is a document approximately 25 to 35 pages in length that specifies the quality management system of an organization. It provides consistent information, both internally and externally, about the organization's quality management system and how the healthcare organization intends to comply with the requirements in the ISO 9001:2000 standard. The quality manual must include:

- The scope of the quality management system

- Documented procedures or reference to them

- A description of the interaction between the processes of the quality management system

The *quality manual* must first define and detail the scope of the quality management system. This quality management system can be defined as, *what my organization*

IMPLEMENTATION GUIDANCE NOTE

The scope of the quality management system should be clearly stated; for example, whether it applies to the whole organization, a number of sections, a unit, or a single section. It should include the organizational structures, responsibilities and authorities, procedures, processes, and resources needed to ensure that the healthcare delivery is of the desired quality; that is, the quality management system should address all factors affecting the quality of the relevant service it provides.

---

does and how. A quality management system is the management structure and systems that control and direct the healthcare organization with regard to quality.

The quality manual should also include or make reference to the corresponding quality system procedures. In lieu of actually incorporating systemwide procedures within the quality manual itself, the ISO 9001:2000 standard allows the organization to make reference to such system procedures either in the quality manual itself or in external documents referenced by the quality manual.

Next, the quality manual or system procedures should include and define the interaction between the processes of the quality management system. Normally these process interactions are described in the quality manual, system procedures, or in policies, work instructions, protocols, and so on. Healthcare organizations traditionally call work instructions *protocols* or *how-to* documents. Figure 3.1 is an example of the sequence and interaction of a healthcare process found in a typical in vitro fertilization (IVF) clinic. In this example, marketing initiates initial contact with the patient. Once the patient has decided on the services of the IVF clinic, patient financial services registers the patient, schedules the initial consultation with the physician, and schedules required lab workups. A clinical plan (quality plan) is created, treatment provided, and desired outcomes identified. The patient is billed and follow-up is scheduled and carried out. There are many methods that can be used to document a healthcare organization's sequence and interaction of processes.

Figure 3.2 shows a typical hospital sequence and interactions flowchart. The sequence and interaction of process flow begins with public relations and community education. This sequence is followed by administrative planning. Resources are identified and provided by administration, and personnel are trained, qualified, and in some cases, credentialed. The next sequence is registration of patients, provision of care, discharge, billing, and analysis of data gathered throughout the healthcare delivery continuum. After the data is analyzed, it is fed back through the applicable processes to public relations and community relations, so improvements can be made to any processes that appear ineffective. The ISO 9001:2000 standard requires the organization to identify the sequence and interactions within the quality management system as described in the quality manual.

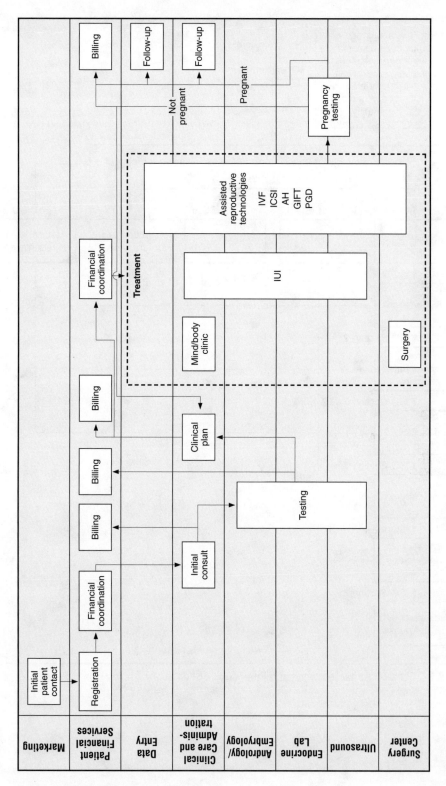

Figure 3.1 Sequence and interaction of a healthcare process.

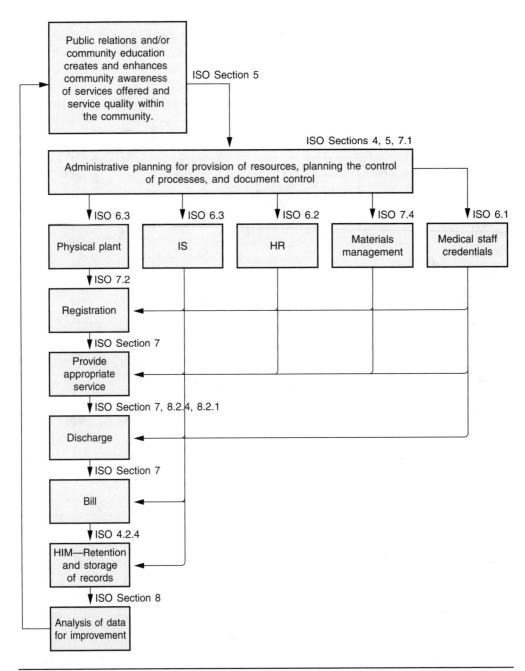

Figure 3.2 Typical hospital sequence and interaction of healthcare processes.

Introduction to the Quality Manual

There are a number of good reasons for having a quality manual. The most compelling reason is that it is a requirement of the ISO 9001 standard. A quality manual will provide:

- A method for defining the healthcare organization's quality policy

- A way to document the quality management structure

- A good management aid for defining employees' responsibilities

- A method for demonstrating management's commitment to quality

- A document that can be used for training purposes

- A useful marketing tool for potential customers (large corporations seeking healthcare delivery contracts with hospitals, clinics, or occupational health clinics)

- A method for providing continuity of the system as personnel change

- A basis for carrying out internal self-assessment audits

Preparation for Writing the Quality Manual

Before writing a quality manual, consider who the end users of the manual will be, as this may dictate both the format and contents of the manual. If the manual is written for a registration/certification body, then it will have to include the specific minimum requirements of the ISO 9001:2000 standard.

The quality manual may also be written to satisfy a patient/customer; if so, their requirements will have to be addressed as well as the requirements of the ISO 9001:2000 standard. Typically, this is not the case within the healthcare field, but it may be necessary in the manufacturing or service sectors.

A healthcare organization may wish to write a quality manual solely to satisfy the needs of its own internal organization and fulfill the requirements of its own quality management system.

There is no defined format for a quality manual. Style and format can be a matter of personal choice. The important thing is that the quality manual addresses the requirements of the quality management system in operation within the healthcare organization. It is useful to follow a structured system with its stated requirements. If the healthcare organization is seeking registration to ISO 9001, then these requirements will have to be addressed in the quality manual (see appendix B, Sample Quality Systems Manual and Procedures).

It is often difficult to decide what to put into the quality manual and what to leave out. Depending on the size of the healthcare organization and the complexity of the operation, it is usually better to have a separate procedures manual (see System-Level Procedures and Sample System-Level Procedures in appendix B). This will contain all the written procedures for operating the quality system. It could also include work instructions, checklists, and training details, or these may be contained in separate manuals. Each procedure or work instruction will be given its own number and will be referenced from the quality manual or a master reference list. This will keep the quality manual compact, neat, and tidy.

Proprietary Information

A healthcare organization may have proprietary information that it does not wish to divulge. This information should be kept separate from the quality manual. This is particularly important if the healthcare organization plans to show its quality manual to patients/customers or competitors. In these circumstances, it may be useful to have an uncontrolled version of the quality manual for information and marketing purposes.

Quality Manual Header Formatting

Each page of the quality manual should have a simple block title header that contains the healthcare organization's logo and basic information. The header identifies the document, when it was issued and revised, and personnel who have reviewed and approved the manual.

| **Quality Paradigms Medical Center** **ISO 9001:2000 Quality Systems Manual** | Quality Systems Manual Page X of XX |
| | Issued: Revised: Supersedes: |

Responsibility for the Quality Manual

It is a requirement of the ISO 9001:2000 standard that a person be designated as a management representative with responsibility and authority for ensuring that the requirements of the quality system and ISO 9001:2000 standard are implemented and maintained. Some organizations have multiple management representatives or a committee that acts as its management representative. This is acceptable as long as there is a coordinated effort between the assigned personnel having appropriate authority and responsibility. Such authority and responsibility should be assigned and documented. It is strongly recommended that one person be assigned this task in lieu of multiple or group management representatives. The responsibility of management representative is usually assigned to the quality manager or risk manager, as part of his or her responsibility would include writing, coordinating, and distributing the quality manual.

In acting as coordinator for the quality manual, the designated representative must have the full cooperation of everyone in the organization who is involved in quality and process-related policies and procedures. Typically, this individual also heads up and oversees the cross-functional team.

Above all, the organization's administrative management must accept the quality manual, and this acceptance must be made known throughout the healthcare organization. This acceptance is generally documented by the top person's signature and date.

Information Gathering

It will be necessary to collect information from various departments relating to the quality system in order to write the quality manual. This is usually accomplished by forming a cross-functional team, comprising various disciplines. This team is often known as the ISO team.

The management representative should talk to the managers in each department, explain what the purpose of the required information is, and ask for their help. The management representative must work with departmental managers in documenting and developing the manual for each area. Having the managers write the details for their areas of responsibility is an excellent way to collect information and get them involved.

Writing the Quality Manual

The quality manual should be written in straightforward simple language using the present tense. Sentences should be short and to the point. It may be tempting to show off one's vocabulary skills, but do not use complex, rarely used words. Highly technical terms should not be used unless they are properly defined and explained in the quality manual. It is often necessary to create a section for terms, definitions, and acronyms.

The quality manual should be as readable as possible. This means writing in a style understood by the majority of people who will read the manual. It is very important that the quality manual be a statement of the activities in operation in the healthcare organization at the time. It should not cover what has been done in the past or what might be done in the future but what is occurring in the present. It must not contain detailed activities that are not being carried out. The manual should not be embellished to make it look good. *The quality manual must be a reflection of the actual quality system.*

The detailed contents of quality manuals will vary considerably between one healthcare organization and another depending on the nature of the operation to be covered (products or services). The contents of the quality manual will also depend on the level of control that will be applied to a particular operation. A quality management system conforming to the requirements of ISO 9001 may run 25 to 35 or more pages.

Contents of the Quality Manual

The quality manual's contents, headings, and topic formats are up to the organization. The following content and topic examples are geared towards the requirements of the ISO 9001 standard since most healthcare organizations will be implementing ISO 9001:2000 in order to be certified. The quality manual may contain the following headings or topics: table of contents, introduction, quality policy statement, revision sheet, distribution list, updating procedures, purpose terminology, organizational data, and quality system requirements.

Table of Contents or Index. The table of contents is self-explanatory and should be compiled on completion of the manual. It is useful to have a clear, logical classification system using numbers or coding. If necessary, the system should be explained in the quality manual or a corresponding system-level procedure.

Introduction. An introduction states that the purpose of the manual is to describe the activities to be conducted for controlling the quality of the product or service carried out by the healthcare organization.

Quality Policy Statement. This can be a very simple statement of the healthcare provider's quality policy detailing the organization's commitment to provide services of the highest quality standard for its customers.

ANSI/ISO/ASQ Q9000-2000 defines *quality policy* as the "overall intentions and direction of an organization related to quality as formally expressed by top management." The quality policy forms one key element of the corporate policy. The quality policy is typically signed by the chief executive, president, or administrator who, by signing, commits to the publication and acceptance of the policies, activities, and systems set forth in the quality manual.

Revision or Amendment Sheet. This sheet is for recording any alterations or changes to the quality manual, ensuring that each manual contains a complete record of all changes. This sheet is typically on the manual's cover page or on an attachment to the manual.

Distribution or Manual Holders List. The distribution list shows the number of manuals in existence and the names of those who have numbered copies. Electronic copies of the manual may allow everyone in the organization to have viewing access. Typically, there is at least one hard copy of the manual even when electronic versions are available.

Procedures for Updating the Manual. This section contains specific instructions for each manual holder as to the procedure to be undertaken to ensure that each copy of the quality manual is kept up-to-date. Any amendments typically are reviewed and approved by the person responsible for the quality manual.

Purpose of the Quality Manual. A narrative purpose statement describes the quality manual as a working document containing the healthcare provider's general overall organizational structure, policies, and activities for achieving and maintaining the quality of its healthcare delivery services. The purpose statement may also describe the quality manual as a source of reference for all matters dealing with quality that can be used by potential customers as a means of assessing the healthcare organization's quality management system.

> **IMPLEMENTATION GUIDANCE NOTE**
>
> The quality manual does not have to be a stand-alone document. It can be a part of a broader-based document covering all aspects of the healthcare organization's activities. It also does not have to be called a quality manual. It can be given whatever title is suitable for the healthcare organization. In some healthcare organizations, the Leadership section of the JCAHO Manual may be deemed the *quality manual,* while in others it may be called the *plan for the provision of care.* In either case, modification to the existing documents will need to be implemented or cross-reference documents created to identify where currently established requirements are consistent with ISO 9001:2000 requirements.

Definitions and Terminology. It may be necessary to provide a list of definitions and terms used in the manual so readers have a clear and complete understanding of its contents. This is particularly true when terms peculiar to the healthcare organization are used. ISO 9000-2000 is a useful reference for additional vocabulary and terms.

Organizational Data. Since the quality manual may be given to customers, this page gives general details about the healthcare organization:

- Name, health system, subsidiaries, clinics, labs, and so on
- Scope of services provided
- Number of staff
- Location

Quality Manual and the Quality System Requirements. The previous sections of the quality manual are of an introductory and general nature. The quality manual need not contain all of the previous information but it is useful. The body of the manual is the nuts and bolts of the quality management system. The main sections will, out of necessity, be the longest in the manual. The length and content will vary according to the size of the organization, methods of operation, the kind of quality program, and the type of product or service provided.

QUALITY SYSTEM LEVEL PROCEDURES AND DOCUMENTATION

The ISO 9001:2000 standard requires the creation and use of *procedures.* Healthcare organizations that are accredited by different accrediting bodies are not new to the concept of writing policies and procedures. Procedures within the ISO 9001:2000 scheme are different than those mandated by accreditation bodies. ISO 9001:2000 procedures are used to ensure that organizational processes and their interactions are defined. By documenting the way processes operate within the framework of the healthcare organization, improvement within those processes may take place as personnel discover new and improved ways of carrying out defined tasks. The ISO 9001:2000 term *procedure* (specified way to carry out an activity or process) causes some bewilderment when implementing a quality management system within healthcare organizations because typically procedures are referred to as *policies and procedures.* The term *procedure* standing alone often causes confusion to those working within the organization.

Quality system procedures are documents that describe how the quality management system is applied to a specific product, service, project, or contract. These documents may also be referred to as *quality plans.* Additionally, quality system procedures specify the ways to carry out an activity or a process.

ISO 9001:2000, Subclause 4.2.1 identifies several different requirements in which documented procedures must be created or established. As stated, there are six system-level required procedures identified in the ISO 9001:2000 standard:

- 4.2.3 Control of documents

- 4.2.4 Control of records

- 8.2.2 Internal audit

- 8.3 Control of nonconforming product

- 8.5.2 Corrective action

- 8.5.3 Preventive action

Additionally, procedures are required when such procedures are needed by the healthcare organization to ensure effective planning, operation, and control of the service delivery processes.

The ISO 9001:2000 standard does not specify any specific format when creating and drafting procedures. The procedure format is the healthcare organization's choice, but the scope of the documented management system will need to address each of the ISO 9001:2000 requirements. When drafting quality system procedures, the format should keep the documentation structure organized, complete, easy to understand, and carefully identified.

Many times healthcare organizations ask, "How much documentation do I need to generate?" ISO 9001:2000 Subclause 4.2.1 Note 2 states that the amount of your organization's documentation depends on three factors.

The Size and Type of Activities That Are a Part of the Organization

If a healthcare organization is small, with simple or redundant activities, practices, and processes, the amount of documentation required may be minimal. If the healthcare organization is a large, multisite, multifunctioned organization, a large amount of documentation may be necessary to apply effective control over operational processes.

The Complexity of the Processes and Their Interactions

Complex processes will always require more detailed procedures. Simple processes may not require the same level of detail as those with greater complexity. Therefore, the more complex an organization is, the greater the requirement for additional detailed documentation.

The Competence of Personnel

Healthcare organizations where processes and activities are not complex and where a high degree of employee competency, training, and education exists may not require copious amounts of detailed procedures or instructions. Healthcare organizations where processes and activities are complex and where a high degree of competency, training, and education does not exist may require many detailed procedures or instructions.

The nature and extent of the documentation should satisfy the contractual, statutory, and regulatory requirements as well as the needs and expectations of patients/customers. Lengthy written procedures are rarely read thoroughly—if at all! Keep procedures simple and easy to understand.

RULES FOR WRITING PROCEDURES

Procedures describe the way a particular activity or process is to be carried out. Procedures should address and answer the following questions:

How is an activity carried out?

Who is responsible for each aspect of the activity?

What records need to be collected and maintained?

Where is the activity carried out?

When should the activity be carried out?

Why is the activity carried out?

When writing procedures, remember the four rules of procedure writing:

1. Decide what you want to say.

2. Decide how you are going to say it.

3. Use simple, clear language.

4. Keeping the readers in mind will determine the style of writing.

The art of procedure writing lies in making it neither too long nor too short; it should be brief but complete. A procedure should contain sufficient information to allow a newcomer to carry out a process activity without having to seek detailed guidance from colleagues.

Another general rule is that any procedure should be explained in three to seven pages plus attachments. If a procedure is longer than this, you may need to consider whether it should be more than one procedure or one procedure plus a supplementary work instruction.

Procedure Writing Format

It is recommended that written procedures be presented in a standardized format. This has three advantages:

1. It assists the person writing the procedure to identify *what* information needs to be included and *where* it should be included.

2. It helps readers find information quickly and easily, rather than having to search for it.

3. It gives internal quality auditors conducting self-assessments and third-party registration auditors or surveyors confidence that there is a disciplined and structured approach to the organization's documentation.

The format used does not matter; what is important is that it is standardized. The following example illustrates a standardized format that is an industrywide *best practice* format. Each paragraph heading is in bold punctuated with a colon, and followed by text.

A typical procedure must contain the following seven paragraph headings. After each heading, there is a brief summary of the procedure topic.

Purpose: The first paragraph of the procedure must identify the purpose of the procedure in specific terms (aims). The purpose relates what the procedure will cover, the depth of coverage, and general information about how the procedure will be used.

Scope: The second paragraph contains the scope of the procedure (where the procedure's boundaries lie). Any exclusions or limitations should also be stated.

References or Related Documents: Although not necessary, the procedure should identify and list any regulations, standards, or specifications that are referred to in the procedure. Additionally, any needed supplementary procedures or work instructions should be listed.

Definitions: In this section, any positions that have specific responsibilities within the procedure should be identified. Any words, terms, or abbreviations with special significance should also be defined here.

Procedure Method or Process: This section should state how a particular process, practice, or activity should be carried out. This section of the procedure should state in detail the actions necessary to achieve the aims defined in the purpose and scope of the procedure format.

The actual text in the procedure should describe the sequence of actions and inter-actions of the process or activity. The procedure, method, or process description should be brief but include the following:

- Information necessary to perform or carry out the process or task described in the procedure

- The end result from implementing the process or task defined in the procedure

- The responsibilities and duties of people undertaking tasks, processes, and activities described in the procedure

- The method by which customer requirements are to be met

- The specific quality checks used to monitor the tasks, processes, and activities described in the procedure

- The specific records necessary to demonstrate that the essential tasks, processes, and activities of the procedure have been correctly undertaken

- *What-if* actions that may need to be taken and the way to deal with any nonconformances as a result of carrying out the tasks, processes, or activities

- Supporting documentation that is generated and any records that have to be kept

It may also be necessary to describe in the procedure why the task, activity, or process should be carried out in a particular manner. This is especially true if there is specific reason for using the *one best* method from a variety of possible alternatives.

Records: While not required, this section may identify any records that are to be retained as evidence that the task, activity, or process has been completed as an assurance of quality. It may also define the time line for retention of the records.

Attachments: Flowcharts, illustrations, sample forms, and so on, may be included as attachments.

THE QUALITY PLAN

The Clause 7 Product realization section of ISO 9001:2000 refers to a *quality plan*. ANSI/ISO/ASQ Q9000-2000 defines a quality plan as, "a document specifying which procedures and associated resources shall be applied, by whom, and when to a specific project, product, process or contract."

The quality plan usually references the parts of a quality manual, procedures, or work instructions and describes how a specific process, activity, or task is carried out in order to achieve a planned outcome for a predetermined measure of quality. Quality plan documents are generally the output of the planning process.

WRITING HOW-TO DOCUMENTS: WORK INSTRUCTIONS AND PROTOCOLS

ISO 9001:2000 requires that written work instructions, when deemed necessary by the organization, be available. Work instructions are documents defined by the healthcare organization necessary for carrying out detailed work activities. Work instructions provide users with more detailed information than procedures about *how* to perform tasks and activities. Work instructions may be in the form of protocols, books, how-to documents, work flows, flowcharts, and so on.

Subclause 7.5.1 states that when carrying out service delivery processes, such processes must be carried out under controlled conditions. The standard goes on to state that "controlled conditions shall include, as applicable . . . b) the availability of work instructions . . ." It is important to note that the standard *does not* require the creation of work instructions but specifically states that they will be used *as applicable.* Therefore, it is up to the healthcare organization to use or not use work instructions.

4.2.1(E) RECORDS REQUIRED

ANSI/ISO/ASQ Q9000-2000 defines a record as "a document stating results achieved or providing evidence of activities performed." Some of the purposes of records include, but are not limited to, these purposes:

- Providing evidence that specified requirements have been met

- Providing traceability to products or services that were rendered

- Facilitating appropriate preventive and corrective actions

ISO 9001:2000 Subclause 4.2.4 provides additional requirements and more detailed information for control of records.

4.2.3 CONTROL OF DOCUMENTS

A healthcare organization should establish and identify what documents and data it must maintain control over. Controlled documents should suit the healthcare organization's method and scope of operation. Document control applies to all documents and data in the form of hard copy, electronic, or other media. Documents used to define, direct, and control activities that affect the healthcare organization's quality management system should be placed under document control.

During a recent evaluation of a hospital that was readying itself to implement ISO 9001:2000, the writer noted that the *consent forms* and *Medicare reimbursement* forms signed by patients during the admission process in the past year appeared to contain outdated information. Upon further investigation, more recent versions of the forms were found in the hospital print shop. Admissions had been using the outdated forms for more than six months! What potential risk was the hospital exposed to as a result of this error? How many more forms used within the organization were out of date that may have led to patient safety concerns or other professional liability or compliance issues?

The primary purpose for the control of documents is to ensure that all necessary, accurate, and up-to-date manuals, procedures, policies, protocols, and forms are available to those who need them. Document control covers the creation, distribution, and retention of internal documents and the receipt, distribution, and retention of external documents that have an affect on the quality management system and the quality of healthcare delivery, programs, and services.

As control of documents is one of the six procedures required by ISO 9001:2000, the procedure must describe and address the following:

- The controls used for approval and review of documents prior to their distribution

- The process used to update, change, and approve documents

- Identification of documents (issue number, revision status, issue date)

- The controls used to distribute and retrieve obsolete documents

- The process and controls necessary to ensure that documents are available where activities affecting service delivery are carried out

- The control and distribution of documents received from outside of the organization

There can be some difficulty in deciding the difference between a document and a record. A simple rule of thumb is that a document can be revised, whereas a record cannot. For example, a quality manual can be revised and is controlled by ISO 9001:2000 Subclause 4.2.3, Control of documents, while a patient's medical record cannot be revised. The medical record is controlled in accordance with the requirements specified in ISO 9001:2000 Subclause 4.2.4 Control of records.

Examples of typical documents for which control should be considered include the following:

- The quality manual

- System-level procedures, policies, and procedures

- Protocols and instructions

- Work instructions

- List of approved subcontractors including casual staff

- Statements of regulatory requirements

- Policies and reference to requirements or external manuals such as health department or national standards, schedule forms, and treatment program information

- Computer software used to control, measure, or monitor processes and manuals

- Catalogues and similar patient/client literature

The healthcare organization should develop a method for ensuring that these documents are available to staff. Only current versions of the management system documents should be available, and a means of identifying and withdrawing superseded documents should be documented within the procedure.

The method of document control may vary according to the type of document. For example, critical procedures such as infection control, surgery, and anesthesia procedures need a tightly controlled system; whereas a list of approved vendors might be circulated against an approved distribution list.

The type of control and records needed to control documentation may vary according to the type and criticality of the document. For the quality manual, policies and procedures, protocols, books and instructions, a formal system of numbered documents and controlled issue for who holds and maintains documents might be considered.

A less rigid control might be considered for other written materials that are distributed according to an approved distribution list. External documents such as forms, manuals, regulations, statutes, and standards from external bodies need to be kept up-to-date and may need to be registered or issued through a library (see the following section, Control of Documents of External Origin).

A healthcare organization should adopt a document control system that suits its method and mode of operation. Where the healthcare organization finds it necessary to change a document, the documentation control procedure should document and identify the change control methodology and who is responsible for review and approval of changes.

FORMS CONTROL

Each organization uses forms in its day-to-day operations of management systems. Forms are used to document that specific requirements have been met. Forms must be controlled and their approval documented.

Forms should not be confused with records. Blank forms are considered documents and must be controlled as such in accordance with the requirements of ISO 9001:2000 Subclause 4.2.3. Forms should be carefully evaluated. Over time, forms tend to proliferate and become redundant or obsolete. While recently developing ISO 9001:2000 quality management systems, several hospitals decreased the number of forms being used by as many as 1000. Controls must ensure that the current forms are being used and that obsolete forms are promptly removed from use.

CONTROL OF DOCUMENTS OF EXTERNAL ORIGIN

Documents that may not be included in the quality manual but are listed as *referenced documents* are sometimes referred to as documents of external origin. These documents must be identified and their distribution controlled. Such documents may include the following:

- The rights and responsibilities of patients/customers

- Accredited programs or services (JCAHO, CAP, CLIA)

- References to professional and other external bodies

- References to safety and emergency procedures

- Professional books, handbooks, Joint Commission, or CAP standards

- Government policies, regulations, and administrative books (CMA, Conditions of Participation, CLIA, FDA, DEA)

- Electronic medical records (EMR) computer software programs and their revisions (MEDITECH, MediNotes Charting Plus, SmartClinic)

Documents of an external nature that are used within the healthcare organization to carry out service delivery or that are used to control service delivery must be identified in a suitable manner. Additionally, when distributing or installing external documents, their whereabouts must be known at all times in order to facilitate recall of the documents when external parties revise and reissue them.

4.2.4 CONTROL OF RECORDS

Healthcare organizations should control any records and documents that the organization is required to maintain to meet legal and statutory obligations and other records generated as a result of the service delivery process. These include patient records (hard copy or EMR), admission and discharge records (hard copy or EMR), drug registers, goods receipts, and so forth. During several consulting contracts involving a wide array of healthcare organizations, it was noted that there were typically no documented procedures regarding the identification, indexing, filing, and retention times of records. This may be a missing element within many healthcare organizations.

In addition to these requirements, a number of clauses in the ISO 9001:2000 standard refer to specific requirements for record keeping. Most healthcare service organizations have an established system for maintaining records and therefore should begin by reviewing existing procedures against the requirements of Subclause 4.2.4, only adding or simplifying existing procedures where appropriate.

Establishment of the quality system should not result in unnecessary paperwork or duplication of records, and the first step in assessing this should be an evaluation of existing records and the effectiveness of existing record-keeping procedures.

Archiving and retrieval procedures, retention times, provisions for access to, and methods of disposal for records should be set down in the records control procedure.

Where records are kept electronically, procedures may need to consider systems for archiving, maintaining software needed to access old records, backing up, and storing electronic media such as computer disks.

The bottom line is that records must be identified, indexed, filed, stored, and disposed of in accordance with the healthcare organization's documented procedures.

In summary, the healthcare organization must document its management system, address each ISO 9001:2000 requirement, and arrange information in an orderly manner. This leaves much flexibility for building a quality management system that meets both business needs and the needs and expectations of customers. The structure of the organization's documentation must be crafted in a manner that works for the healthcare organization.

There are many ways of accomplishing the intent of the ISO 9001:2000 standard, and the healthcare organization should adopt those approaches that best suit its mode of operation. The healthcare organization should verify that the implementation approaches defined in this book provide for an effective quality management system. Each healthcare organization should identify its key processes by building on its existing policies and procedures and management control systems to develop an effective quality management system suitable for, and structured to reflect, the scope of services it supplies and the processes and specific practices it employs.

ENDNOTES

1. Documents: information and its supporting medium. A *document* is defined as, but not limited to, a *record, specification, procedure document, drawing, report,* or *standard.* A set of documents is frequently called *documentation.* The supporting medium can be paper, magnetic, electronic, optical computer disk, photograph, master sample, or a combination thereof. ANSI/ISO/ASQ Q9000-2000.

4

ISO 9001:2000 Clause 5—Management Responsibility

Leadership: healthcare leaders establish unity of purpose, direction, and internal environment of the healthcare organization. Leadership creates the environment in which people can become fully involved in achieving the healthcare organization's objectives. Everything rises and falls on leadership!

5.1 MANAGEMENT COMMITMENT

Executive management or administration maintains the sole responsibility for defining and documenting organizational responsibilities for quality and for ensuring that the goals, objectives, and commitment for quality care are met throughout the organization. The executive management must ensure that the quality management system is implemented effectively throughout the entire organization (not just clinical) to enhance patient/customer satisfaction. This commitment will enhance continual improvement throughout the service delivery process. Organizational priorities that relate to enhancing the service provided and improving patient outcomes are critical components in the delivery of healthcare services. Management must ensure that all provided services meet the defined and documented quality policy, goals, and objectives, bringing about effective quality management and continual improvement.

5.2 CUSTOMER FOCUS

Top management or administration must demonstrate and ensure that customer requirements are being met with the aim of enhancing customer satisfaction. The healthcare organization must identify suitable methods to determine and verify that patient/customer needs and expectations are being met in order to enhance their satisfaction. This determination and verification will most likely be identified during the implementation of ISO 9001:2000 Subclause 7.2 Customer-related processes and Subclause 8.2.1 Customer satisfaction.

Top management or administration must establish that personnel have the necessary skills and competency, what patient/customer needs and expectations are, and that the organization has the capability to meet those needs.

CUSTOMER FOCUS—WHO IS THE CUSTOMER?

The ultimate goal of any continual improvement effort is to better understand and then satisfy the needs of the patient/customer. Thus, before formulating any continual improvement goals or strategic targets, the healthcare organization must first assess who its customers are. Focusing on customers will raise fundamental questions about the purpose and mission of the healthcare organization. When identifying customers, the healthcare organization should ask the following eight questions from Dr. Deming to assist in stimulating thinking about patients/customers:

1. Who makes decisions about purchasing your healthcare-related service or product?

2. How do you distinguish between *quality* as your customer perceives it and *quality* as the healthcare organization's staff and leaders perceive it?

3. How does the quality of the service delivery, as the customer sees it, agree with the quality that the organization intends to provide?

4. Do the organization's patients/customers think that the service delivery lives up to their expectations?

5. What does the healthcare organization know about the problems of patients/customers in the use of the service that was delivered?

6. Does the healthcare organization depend on complaints from customers to learn what is wrong with the service?

7. Are patients/customers satisfied with the service delivery that is provided? If they are, what is satisfactory about it? How is that known?

8. Will the organization's patients/customers of today be patients/customers a year in the future? Two years in the future?

Information concerning patients/customers can be gathered from a large number of sources. One method of identifying patient/customer requirements is to gather a cross-functional team of different department personnel and complete a *customer affinity diagram*. Since most healthcare organizations have many different patients/customers, it is typical for them to separate patients/customers into smaller subgroups, often referred to

---

IMPLEMENTATION GUIDANCE NOTE

In many cases, patient/customer needs (what they want) and expectations (what they expect to receive) are not the same. For example, a patient may expect a particular outcome for a medical condition. However, this expectation may be beyond the capability of current medical interventions and/or knowledge. Do not ignore this point. How has the healthcare organization communicated this to the patient/customer?

---

as *customer segments*. Most healthcare organizations segment patient/customers based on what products and/or services they use. Patient/customer segmentation assists in defining the requirements of different populations. Segmentation also provides a sampling basis for understanding similarities among patients/customers. Additionally, segmentation clarifies which patient/customer groups can be impacted by improvement efforts focused on a particular service.

5.3 QUALITY POLICY

The healthcare organization must have a documented quality policy that clearly reflects its mission, vision, goals, and objectives The quality policy should take into account the requirements and expectations of its patients and other customers. The quality policy must include some element of continual improvement.

The healthcare organization should establish how it will communicate the quality policy to its staff. Methods for such communication could include staff meetings, orientation sessions, workshops, health fairs, job fairs, training sessions, e-mail, intranet sites, pay stubs, posters, bulletin boards, wallet-sized cards, and so on. All personnel must understand their role in implementing the quality policy as well as meeting the organization's stated mission, values, goals, and objectives. One important aspect of communicating the quality policy is ensuring that all staff members understand the organization's goals and objectives relating to the needs and expectations of patients/customers as well as the community at large. Patients/customers should be made aware of the organization's quality policy, values, and objectives.

The quality policy must be reviewed periodically by top management or administration and should reflect changes in organizational tasks, processes, activities, and the changing needs and expectations of patients/customers.

5.4 PLANNING

Planning within the quality management system typically includes plans that establish quality objectives, processes to be employed by the organization, and methods for measuring and monitoring system performance.

IMPLEMENTATION GUIDANCE NOTE

The quality policy may already exist as part of the healthcare provider's current strategic planning process or corporate mission/vision statements. This is not uncommon in the healthcare industry. Typically the healthcare provider will define, document, and publish a mission statement or similar statement of vision, purpose, or commitment. Healthcare organizations sometimes choose to initiate an organizationwide mission or vision statement independent of their quality system aspirations. Provided that there are measurable elements to such statements, and that these statements reflect the requirements in ISO 9001:2000 Subclause 5.3, then these statements may be used in lieu of the ISO quality policy.

IMPLEMENTATION GUIDANCE NOTE

The following table may be used when evaluating the organization's quality policy and objectives. The quality policy and objectives should be established to provide evidence of an organizational focus and added direction throughout the entire healthcare organization.

Quality Policy

Defined: Overall intentions and direction of an organization related to quality as formally expressed by top management.

Is the quality policy consistent with the overall policy of the organization?

Does the policy provide a framework for establishing and setting quality objectives?

Does the policy provide a framework for reviewing quality objectives?

Does the quality policy identify the commitment of management to meet requirements?

Does the policy establish a commitment for continual improvement?

Is the policy communicated throughout the organization and is it understood?

Is the policy reviewed for continuing suitability?

Quality Objectives

Defined: Something sought or aimed for, relating to quality.

Are objectives based on the organization's quality policy?

Are objectives specified for various functions and levels within the organization?

Are objectives consistent with the quality policy?

Objectives demonstrate a commitment to continual improvement?

Is achievement of objectives measurable?

Does achievement of objectives provide a positive impact on service delivery, operational effectiveness, and financial performance?

Does achievement of objectives provide a positive impact on the satisfaction and confidence of patients/customers?

There are many planning tools in use today by management, and one of the most popular is hoshin planning. Hoshin planning is used through an organizationwide process where a vision is created and action is taken. *Hoshin* is derived from the Japanese, *hoshin kanri,* which means *policy deployment.* The healthcare organization formulates a plan, transforms action plan inputs into measurable plan outputs or results, and then measures and monitors the effectiveness of the plan. Any planning, regardless of the methods used, should include topics regarding continual improvement, process improvement, and enhanced customer satisfaction.

5.4.1 QUALITY OBJECTIVES

In order to implement an effective quality policy, top management or administration will need to establish quality goals and objectives within the organization. These objectives may relate to the quality management system and its improvement as well as relating to those products and/or services that are provided by the healthcare organization.

Quality objectives need to be realistic and must have some measurable component. The healthcare organization achieves and carries out its objectives as it provides day-to-day care to patients/customers.

The achievement of objectives is measured through the evaluation and monitoring of healthcare delivery processes. As processes are measured and monitored, objectives are evaluated as to their effectiveness to meet requirements; objectives should be amended or new objectives developed based on the measuring and monitoring results.

IMPLEMENTATION GUIDANCE NOTE

While evaluating the healthcare organization's quality goals and objectives, top management shall ensure that the objectives created by the healthcare organization are SMART objectives:

Specific   Objectives must be *specific* and relate to the quality policy.

Measurable   Objectives must have some *measurable* components.

Attainable   Objectives that need to be *attained* must be within the organization's reach.

Reasonable   Objectives must be *reasonable* and contain logic.

Timely   Objectives must have a defined *time* frame.

It is common to find departmental goals and objectives defined in larger healthcare provider facilities. In those cases, each departmental manager and/or director provides yearly continuous quality improvement (CQI) plans that often include departmental objectives. Such departmental objectives must be in line with corporate initiatives, goals, and objectives.

5.4.2 QUALITY MANAGEMENT SYSTEM PLANNING

The healthcare organization must be able to demonstrate that organizational planning activities have been conducted and performed. Such planning activities establish the means by which the requirements for quality will be met. Quality system documentation such as procedures, policies and procedures, and protocols may fully satisfy the quality management system planning requirements. Planning should also include how the quality and service delivery requirements for a particular service scope will be met and how clinical inputs (diagnosis), clinical care (interventions), and outcomes (response to treatment) will be verified or evaluated. Such planning may be required both strategically and operationally.

Strategic planning, for example, may include planning a new scope of service that will be offered, identifying what treatment would be provided, and allocating adequate resources to support the new service. Strategic planning may involve input from the community at large, customer feedback, changing demographics of the area such as an increasing or decreasing population, and other consumer groups.

Operational planning may include the setting out of the specific practices, resources, and sequence of processes and activities relevant to the particular healthcare service, project, or contract offering. These specifics would go in a planning document or other documented procedures.

Quality management system planning should also cover both clinical and nonclinical processes within the management system. The planning documents and records of planning must demonstrate and identify how objectives will be achieved. Too often healthcare organizations focus primarily on clinical outcomes and forget that planning the supporting nonclinical areas is as critical.

Planning output documents should be in a format that fits the needs of the healthcare organization, and personnel need to be familiar with these documents. For standard clinical activities, planning may be achieved through the use of existing policies and procedures or by developing training programs. Management system plans can be as

---

IMPLEMENTATION GUIDANCE NOTE

Documents or activities that demonstrate effective quality management system planning include: strategic business plans; quality objectives for a specific activity or systemwide activities; CQI plans and meeting minutes; minutes from planning meetings; the design, delivery, and evaluation of protocols, policies and procedures, and processes to ensure that practice is feasible and integrated within the system; design and development of nursing care plans; resources facilities infrastructure procedures tests, examinations, or patient outcome standards; establishing and documenting thresholds; patient charts and the documenting of patient assessments; measuring and monitoring of care plans at appropriate stages during the patient stay.

brief as a checklist or a work flow that references other parts of the management system. For new activities, services, or processes, the development of a specific planning document, procedure, or manual may be necessary. The processes included in this document can then be adopted as standard policy or procedure once the activity is firmly established (see also 7.1 Planning of product realization).

5.5 RESPONSIBILITY, AUTHORITY AND COMMUNICATION
5.5.1 RESPONSIBILITY AND AUTHORITY

The healthcare provider should identify and define what activities, tasks, and duties personnel are expected to perform (responsibility) and what decisions they can make (authority). This can be communicated with an organization chart, with a job description, or in the quality manual and procedures. Functional areas of responsibility and authority within the organization can be shown on the organization chart. These charts may also identify lines of communication (see 5.5.3 Internal communication). Organization charts can also specify accountability. Alternatively, responsibilities, authorities, and accountabilities (and communication paths) may be described in the quality manual or other procedures.

5.5.2 MANAGEMENT REPRESENTATIVE

The management representative is selected by top management or administration to oversee the ISO 9001:2000 quality management system, to report on its effectiveness, and to communicate the importance of meeting customer requirements to all employees (see 5.5.3 Internal communication). The management representative may work full-time in the area of quality or have other functions or responsibilities; the authority referred to in ISO 9001:2000 Subclause 5.5.1 applies when acting in the role of management representative. The ISO 9001:2000 standard requires that the appointed management representative be a member of management. This appointment is very important as the management representative must have the respect and equality of his or her peers to carry out the duties of implementing the management system. The representative should report directly to top management.

5.5.3 INTERNAL COMMUNICATION

In many organizations, communication is a great weakness. In implementing an effective quality management system, a useful communication methodology must be implemented. The healthcare organization must maintain an internal communication system that enhances healthcare service delivery processes as well as improving the effectiveness of the quality management system. Electronic communication via intranets, the Internet, and e-mail provides an effective and flexible approach. Other methods such as memoranda, postings on bulletin boards, and staff meetings also have a place in this process.

5.6 MANAGEMENT REVIEW

ISO 9001:2000 requires top management or administration to review the effectiveness of the quality management system at regular intervals. Records of management review must be maintained and must demonstrate any actions considered necessary regarding the quality management system, what action was undertaken, and its effectiveness. Management review is conducted to evaluate the health and vitality of the documented management system at defined intervals.

The frequency and depth of management reviews should be in line with the quality management system and the associated risk identified within each part of the healthcare organization as well as within the quality management system.

Management should review the effectiveness of the quality management system as a whole at least once a year. More frequent and detailed attention should be applied to critical areas and to areas where significant changes are planned.

Management review is an evaluation of organizational systemwide processes, practices, methods, and tasks at the strategic level rather than the day-to-day operational level. It should, for example, include review of organizational policies, organizational priorities, success in the achievement of quality objectives, changes within the quality management system, and allocation of capital and other resources.

Many ISO 9001:2000 accredited surveying bodies (registrars) require organizations to have completed at least one cycle of management reviews prior to the registration survey (assessment).

5.6.2 REVIEW INPUT

In many healthcare organizations, committees carry out weekly or monthly reviews of certain operations. These reviews are *not* considered management review. The nature of these meetings is focused around daily operational activities and problems and not on the entire quality management system. While these meetings are no doubt useful, the information that is gathered may or may not be needed during the management review. Findings and recommendations of such committee reviews may become an input into the management review process in the same way the findings from internal self-assessment audits become an input into the management review. Top management or administration should ensure that it has not confused internal audits with management review (see 8.2.2 Internal audit). In addition to the items already mentioned, these other activities should be considered during management review:

- Review of the quality management system's suitability and effectiveness in achieving objectives for quality

- Progress toward the organization's strategic, operational, business, and performance objectives

- Changes to legislation or statutory regulations that may affect the healthcare organization's activities

- Analysis of data and trends in clinical indicators, thresholds, and healthcare outcomes

- Customer feedback including complaints, suggestions, and reports

- External reviews by JCAHO, CMA, CAP, CLIA, AOA, state, and other organizations

- Second and third-party audit reports including internal quality audits and surveys

- Quality improvement, CQI reports, and dashboard indicators including reports from the management representative

- Nonconformities and corrective and preventive action reports

- Training and competency needs and the organization's need for competent, qualified personnel

- Changes to operational methodology and personnel

- Performance of vendors and suppliers

5.6.3 REVIEW OUTPUT

The effect of any changes identified at a previous management review should be assessed. Additional action may be required if the changes did not achieve the desired effect. During the management review, the opportunity for justifiable improvement should be sought and implemented, resources permitting.

In addition to the items already mentioned, outputs to management review should include decisions and actions related to:

- Improvement of the documented management system

- Improvement of its organizational processes

- Improvement of the service delivery processes

- Improved customer satisfaction

- Resource needs

RECORDS OF MANAGEMENT REVIEW

The management representative shall ensure that records of management review are maintained. These records could be minutes of a formal management review meeting or a report summarizing the key issues and actions to be implemented as a result of management review. A memo summarizing issues and actions to be taken may also be provided as a record of management review. Any actions arising from management review must be followed up on. The surveyor (registrar) will be looking for follow-up action during surveillance.

5

ISO 9001:2000 Clause 6— Resource Management

Involvement of people: an organization is comprised of people. The healthcare organization achieves maximum benefit when employees are fully involved, using their abilities to the organization's greatest advantage.

6.1 PROVISION OF RESOURCES

Top management or administration must ensure that adequate resources are available. This provision is typically accomplished through a budgeting and review process.

6.2 HUMAN RESOURCES

The skills, training, education, and competence of all personnel including support staff and care providers in healthcare organizations has a direct bearing on the quality and positive outcome of patient care. Both clinical and nonclinical personnel play a significant part in creating patient /customer expectations and perceptions of the care received. Therefore, the level of qualifications and training required for all personnel performing activities affecting quality needs to be identified and carried out.

Human resources, as used by ISO 9001:2000, includes the management of human resource and the need to communicate to all staff members an awareness of the organization's quality policy and objectives. This includes creating an awareness of their roles in meeting the organization's values and objectives for patient care, both individually and as part of a team.

Records of personnel training, education, qualifications, and details of responsibility and authority specified in position or job descriptions can be developed to complement other quality documentation and records. These records are normally part of human resources files and can form an important part of the quality management system.

When creating human resource documentation, a healthcare organization should review the job or position description and compare it to the experience, qualifications, knowledge, and skills of assigned staff. Records of competency, training, and education must be available and maintained.

Training records should be available for activities such as, but not limited to, the following:

- ISO 9001:2000 management system training

- Internal self-assessment (audit) training

- Safety and emergency procedures

- Compliance issues

- Healthcare skills and knowledge

- Communication skills

- Management skills and knowledge

- Technical or skill-related knowledge

- Quality management skills and knowledge

- Occupational health and workplace safety procedures

- Attendance at conferences, seminars and similar programs

- Opportunity for formal study

- Structured on-the-job training

6.3 INFRASTRUCTURE AND 6.4 WORK ENVIRONMENT

These two subclauses of the ISO 9001:2000 standard address requirements relating to the organization's physical facilities that control the internal environment.

One important attribute of infrastructure is the maintenance of plant equipment. A preventive maintenance system needs to be identified and maintained.

During recent consulting projects in several hospitals, some biomedical and facilities management personnel did not understand the difference between *calibration of equipment* and *preventive maintenance of equipment*. For example, in five hospitals, fetal monitors had not been calibrated as required by the manufacturer's user manual. This was particularly disturbing since one hospital had just settled a lawsuit regarding a fetal monitor that had failed. Fetal monitors in all evaluated hospitals were found to be logged in to the organization's preventive maintenance system, but they were *not* calibrated as a matter of course per the manufacturer's user manual. In fact, biomed personnel were completely unaware that the manufacturer's user manual addressed five pages of calibration requirements!

In several hospitals, numerous pieces of equipment requiring calibration and preventive maintenance were in use throughout the hospital. This equipment had entered the hospital system, bypassing the normal channels of receiving inspection, log-ins, and the asset management tracking system. External sales personnel had introduced this equipment to staff who were very impressed. The department manager was then offered the use of the equipment on a trial basis. The equipment had completely bypassed the normal equipment entry process and was not listed in the preventive maintenance or calibration system. (Calibration is discussed in Subclause 7.6.)

When it comes to preventive maintenance of equipment, a healthcare organization must pay special attention to ensure that:

- Preventive maintenance of equipment is carried out and documented.

- Electrical checks have been conducted on all electrical equipment in patient care areas.

- Infection control procedures (universal precautions and BBP controls) are adhered to.

- Air exchanges and temperatures in surgical suites are monitored.

- Air filters are changed and maintained.

- Emergency equipment is tested on a regular basis.

- Surgical suite decontamination processes are effective to prevent infection.

The list is endless. It is important to note that these activities are normally referred to by the Joint Commission on Accreditation of Healthcare Organizations as the *environment of care.*

The following chart may be used to define the training, competency, and education requirements of clinical and medical staff.

IMPLEMENTATION GUIDANCE NOTE	
Healthcare organizations qualify physicians and clinical staff using a process known as credentialing and privileging.	
Physician/Clinical Credentialing	**Physician/Clinical Privileging**
Defined: The process of verifying the credentials, license, education, training, experience, competence, health status, and judgment of any medical staff that may be granted clinical privileges.	Defined: Authorization granted by the hospital administration to a practitioner to provide specific patient care services in the organization within defined limits based on an individual practitioner's license, education, training, experience, competence, health status, and judgment.

continued

continued

Methods of Credentialing		Methods of Clinical Privileging	
Core Privileges	**Delineation of Privileges**	**Core Privileges**	**Delineation of Privileges**
The physician's credentials, license, education, training, experience, competence, health status, and judgment are verified, and, after approval, he or she is granted privileges.	The physician's credentials, license, education, training, experience, competence, health status, and judgment are verified by checking references and verifying that the professional has experience in the clinical procedures checked off in each block of the checklist.	Utilizing the hospital's defined scope of service, a minimum core list of medical procedure groupings is created. Privileges are granted based upon the general core categories on the list. Exceptions may be granted based on hospital needs and verification of credentials.	A standard list of common surgical procedures is listed on a standard checklist. The physician indicates what procedures he or she is requesting to perform at the hospital by checking off the appropriate blocks.
Verify:	**Verify:**	**Verify:**	**Verify:**
1) Core credentialing procedure	1) Credentialing procedure	1) Core privilege procedure	1) Delineation of privilege procedure
2) Sample physician records	2) Sample physician records	2) Sample physician records	2) Sample physician records
3) That procedure is being followed	3) That procedure is being followed	3) That procedure is being followed	3) That procedure is being followed
Ease of Use:	**Ease of Use:**	**Ease of Use:**	**Ease of Use:**
Less time-consuming	Time-consuming	Less time-consuming	Time-consuming

6

ISO 9001:2000 Clause 7— Product Realization

Process approach: the healthcare organization's desire is to achieve more efficiency when related resources and activities are managed as a process.

7.1 PLANNING OF PRODUCT REALIZATION

Healthcare organizations often both produce tangible products and deliver healthcare services. The ISO standard makes no attempt to translate itself for service industries; the organization applying the standard is responsible for knowing what its products are and for understanding that the term *product* can represent both goods and services, depending on what the organization delivers to its customers.

The previously discussed ISO 9001:2000 Subclause 5.4 Planning focused on the higher-level strategic planning processes: the *who, what,* and *why* of the healthcare organization. Subclause 7.1 Planning of product realization focuses on the detailed operational-level planning that identifies and defines *how, when,* and *where* the delivery of healthcare service will take place. Planning at the operational level should include functional or departmental objectives for each type of service that will be delivered. This level of planning should be consistent with the overall quality policy and objectives defined by top management or administration. In planning how healthcare delivery processes or services will be carried out, the organization must determine:

- Departmental or functional quality objectives and requirements for service delivery

- The need to establish healthcare delivery processes and documents and provide resources specific to the service delivery

- The required verification, validation, monitoring, inspection, and test activities specific to the healthcare service delivery process and the criteria for service acceptance

- The records needed to provide evidence that the healthcare delivery processes and resulting service meet requirements

Once plans have been established and documented, they should be communicated to the appropriate personnel and monitored for compliance. Feedback regarding plan performance should be directed to management since the plans are critical to the ongoing quality management system's effectiveness and enhancement of customer satisfaction.

7.2 CUSTOMER-RELATED PROCESSES

This subclause of the standard requires the healthcare organization to fully understand its patient/customer requirements and have a process in place to review those requirements prior to offering or agreeing to provide services. This review process should be documented and define the review activities *how, when,* and *where.* The review of the patient/customer requirements process must also ensure that assigned personnel verify, prior to commitment to provide the service, that the healthcare organization has the ability and resources to meet the requirements set forth in the agreement.

These agreements exist in healthcare, but are not usually called agreements or contracts, and often are not perceived as relating to customer requirements. The reason for this is that service delivery for healthcare organizations often begins with admission to the facility, where the relationship with the customer (patient) has been until this critical juncture a third-party relationship. The physician has determined what activities are required from the hospital, for example, and the critical communication is from the physician to the hospital even though the patient receives care directly.

To further complicate the issue, payment is typically determined by other parties as well; insurance provider requirements and coverage must be investigated and resolved. All of these concerns are part of the determination and review of requirements that takes place at the time of admission to the healthcare facility. Adding to the complexity of this situation is the element of patient stress as they face activities that are often unknown, often uncomfortable, and in most cases performed in isolation from their supportive loved ones. The goal of any quality management system is to enhance the customer's (patient's) perception of quality, and the challenge here is clear.

The standard's requirements in 7.2 are stated in three separate subclauses: 7.2.1 Determination of requirements related to the product, 7.2.2 Review of requirements related to the product, and 7.2.3 Customer communication.

7.2.2 REVIEW OF REQUIREMENTS RELATED TO THE PRODUCT

This subclause requires an organization to determine all requirements: those specified by the customer, those not stated but necessary, statutes and regulations that apply, and additional requirements from the organization. Continuing the previous example, the admissions associate may need to ask these questions:

- Does this physician's order provide enough information to register this patient?

- Are the dates of service specified on the order?

- Is there any special restriction noted on the doctor's order?

- Does the patient know the schedule for preadmission testing and anesthesia counseling?

- Has the patient been made aware of any restrictions such as fasting prior to surgery?

- Does the patient know when and where to report on the day of surgery?

Patients/customers must be made aware of these and dozens of other issues surrounding their admission. Coordinated communication between the healthcare provider, physician, hospital departments and staff, and the patient/customer is critical in enhancing patient/customer expectations regarding the successful outcome of the services to be delivered.

7.2.2 Review of requirements related to the product requires that requirements be reviewed prior to a commitment to supplying service, ensuring that requirements are defined. Differences between any prior communication and the present one must be resolved. The organization must have has the ability to meet the defined requirements. Records must be maintained and changes documented and communicated to appropriate personnel.

Once all information is gathered, usually at admission, there must be both a review and a record of the review.

Emergency cases may necessitate a different type of review process due to the nature of the emergency services delivered. However, emergencies do not relieve the healthcare organization from the responsibility of reviewing requirements or meeting and enhancing customer satisfaction. The following example shows one hospital emergency room's (ER's) failure to carry out a review of customer requirements prior to commencement of care. Inevitably, each and every time an organization fails to carry out an initial review of patient/customer requirements the end result is an unhappy patient/customer.

During a recent survey (audit), one of the surveyors on the team became ill, so it was decided that a trip to the emergency room was in order. When we arrived, the surveyor described the symptoms to the security person at the front door (the first step in the process). Within minutes, the surveyor was whisked away by a young man in scrubs to have blood drawn and an ultrasound taken. After the blood and ultrasound were taken, the surveyor was instructed to go back to the waiting room and wait. After several wrong turns through confusing hallways, the surveyor made his way back to the security guard's station. While waiting, we pondered what exactly it was that we were waiting for. The only personal information taken was the surveyor's first name. An hour passed, then two, then four, and then six. On numerous occasions during our wait, the surveyor attempted to get information from several different people in the ER only to be told to wait, that someone would be along shortly. After the shift changed, the surveyor did not wish to wait any longer, so we finally left the emergency room.

No one had bothered to create a chart or get any insurance or personal information. No one ever called for the surveyor. No one consulted with the surveyor from the time the blood and ultrasound was taken until we left the ER six hours later. No one seemed concerned about the surveyor or her physical condition, except for the surveyor. The surveyor felt as though she was just another person who filtered in and out of the ER. Somewhere in the hospital, there were several vials of blood and an ultrasound record belonging to a patient, Jane Doe, who was never admitted to the ER. The surveyor had not signed any consent for treatment form even though testing had commenced, nor had anyone reviewed or discussed the surveyors' medical history. It was a complete breakdown of the hospital's ER admission process. The hospital ER personnel failed to determine patient requirements prior to commencing service and failed miserably at meeting or enhancing patient satisfaction. This scenario may occur in some form or another every day in hospital ERs across the country. This problem is a system problem. ISO 9001:2000 was created to solve system problems like this before they cause adverse events. (The Institute of Health reported that 44,000 to 98,000 people die each year as a result of medical errors.) As a happy ending to the story, the surveyor was admitted to her local hospital for surgery two days later. The service was delivered successfully and patient satisfaction enhanced.

The upcoming guidance note describes several clinical and nonclinical activities in which customer requirements are determined and how they are documented.

There can be a difference between what the patient/customer expects at the point of services rendered compared to what the healthcare organization is able to provide, as demonstrated by our scenario. The surveyor expected to walk into the ER, provide admissions with personal information, medical history, and insurance information, be interviewed by a nurse or doctor, wait a short period of time, perhaps have some tests performed, be provided with a diagnosis, a prognosis, and be given treatment, if applicable. None of this ever occurred. Prior to the delivery of service, the healthcare organization must establish with the patient/customer exactly what services are to be provided and how the rendered services will fulfill the customer's needs and meet or exceed expectations.

Some of the typical services offered to patients and other customers within the healthcare setting include preadmission testing, social services, pharmacy services, billing, testing, screening, treatment options, diagnosis, interventions, and probable outcomes. Explanations about how these services will be delivered must be presented to

IMPLEMENTATION GUIDANCE NOTE	
Types of requirements that may be identified include:	
Clinical (Internal Requirements)	**Clinical/Nonclinical (External Requirements)**
Informed consents	Nuclear medicine provider contracts
Anesthesia plans (anesthesia counseling)	EMS contracts
	Food service contracts for other facilities
Advanced directives	
	Laundry service contracts to other facilities
Patient advocate forms	
Physicians orders and discharge orders	Lab service contracts
Consent for treatment	Blood banking
Patient financial responsibility agreements	Physician and other clinical staff contracts

the patient/customer in a clear and concise picture. All marketing literature should be consistent with the products and services that are actually offered by the healthcare organization. Such materials also should be current and up-to-date.

As another example, some patients/customers may enter the healthcare facility alone and may lack the capacity to make decisions on their own or understand requirements. In these cases, certain required documents may not be completed prior to admission or prior to the provision of care in the healthcare facility. When the next of kin is notified or the patient is able to make decisions, these documents will be completed.

In some cases, physician orders may need to be provided and issued verbally. This is an acceptable method of receiving requirements provided there is documented evidence in the medical record or chart that such orders were received, reviewed, and carried out. Additionally, processing of standing orders needs to be described in applicable procedures or protocols. It is important that standing orders remain current and that any changes made to these orders indicate some level of control and acceptance by authorized personnel. Additionally, a documented procedure should be established regarding the carrying out of standing orders.

An issue that is often pertinent to ER admissions is whether the organization has the ability to meet the defined requirements. While not necessarily limited to an ER or to the time of admission, a decision may be made before or during an episode of care that the facility cannot meet the patient's needs. In these cases, the process would define all of the requirements and activities necessary for referring the patient to a more appropriate facility including provision of appropriate transport of the patient to the facility.

7.2.3 CUSTOMER COMMUNICATION

7.2.3 Customer communication requires *effective arrangements* for communicating with customers regarding information about the service provided (product information), handling of enquiries, changes to service, and feedback, especially customer complaints.

In addition to knowing just who the customer is, a healthcare organization must address what customers want and how to measure whether they are getting what they want. Customers' needs and expectations are usually captured through their perceptions and reactions to the use of current services being received. Customers are often concerned only with requirements related to quality of service, cost, and timeliness of service delivery. Communication with patients/customers during the service delivery process is paramount in meeting customer perceptions and in fully satisfying them.

Depending on the healthcare service sector, the organization may choose to provide some type of health information service to its patients/customers. This could be a regular newsletter or information data sheets made available on a need-to-know basis. Additionally, community activities sponsored by the healthcare facility may be advertised via community mailings, public service announcements, newspaper ads, television advertising, social service departments, and so on. According to recent JCAHO patient safety requirements, a healthcare organization should establish communication channels for employees to identify healthcare delivery services that are unacceptable. In fact, some healthcare organizations are required to have a grievance process in place.

Patient/customer communication processes should identify a method to gather satisfaction feedback data. The organization should develop a method for monitoring information related to patient/customer perceptions regarding a healthcare provider's ability to meet requirements.

An effective ISO 9001:2000 management system will assist the organization in defining and carrying out a process to ensure that communication channels are open and working.

7.3 DESIGN AND DEVELOPMENT

In some healthcare organizations, design and/or development of services or plans of care may be applicable; in others, design or development is not.

There has been a great deal of debate on this topic in healthcare facilities that have achieved ISO certification. Some organizations have determined that development of plans of care, treatment plans, and so on, are the responsibility of physicians, who are not members of their facility's staff. In these cases, design and development was excluded from the system. In other cases, physicians are on staff, and their function of determining and/or developing care is clearly within the quality management system. In yet other organizations, routine work was defined as simple process, and the scientific research and development of new treatment methods was determined to be controlled by the ISO requirement of design and development.

If design or development is not applicable, the healthcare organization must exclude this from its quality management system. Exclusions are normally documented in the quality manual with the reasons why design or development activities are not conducted within the scope of service provided by the healthcare organization.

When design and/or development is applicable, the following criteria shall be verified and documented:

- Who is carrying out the work

- What the design and/or development activities are

- The stages in the design and/or development plan and the intermediate steps and activities

- The authorities and responsibilities for each stage or activity

- Design and/or development inputs

- Design and/or development outputs and validation

- Other participating departments, organizations, or support services

- Who is involved when the design and/or development plan changes

This documentation does not need to be elaborate or extensive. In many cases, a simple flowchart may suffice. Where the planning interventions, diagnosis, thresholds, assumptions, or circumstances change, the plan may have to be changed or modified. Such changes should be recorded and require authorization and approval from appropriate personnel.

All personnel involved in planning healthcare design activities should be suitably qualified or experienced to perform the work being undertaken.

For uncomplicated care, nursing care plans may require only one care plan review at the completion of treatment. For very ill patients who require a high degree of complex care, several care plan reviews may be required as patients respond to treatment and new clinical information and patient assessment data becomes available.

Design or development verification is the process of checking the results and outcomes in order to ensure that the nursing care plan conforms to the identified interventions; that is, measuring that the design stage output (interventions) is consistent with the design stage input (diagnosis) and that the patient's condition is either improving or not improving. Care plan design verification is a progressive operation that may be carried out over a number of shifts, days, or even weeks depending on the patient's response to treatment and the complexity of the care plan.

The healthcare organization's design procedure should include details of the verification methodology to be adopted such as who is to carry out design verification and how it is to be performed and documented.

Design validation is the process of confirming (by assessment, observation, and examination) that the patient's expected outcome meets the plan requirements.

IMPLEMENTATION GUIDANCE NOTE			
This is an example of a design and/or development activity applied to a healthcare setting.			
Stage of Design or Development for a Nursing Plan of Care	**Activity**	**Responsibility**	**Record**
Design and development planning	Identify prognosis	Physician	Chart
Design and development inputs	Diagnosis	Physician and nurse	Chart/computer
Design and development outputs	Plan of care and interventions	Nursing staff	Chart/computer
Design and development reviews	Review care plan interventions	Nursing staff	Chart/computer
Design and development verification	Verify effectiveness of interventions (output meets inputs)	Nursing staff	Chart/computer
Design and development validation	Validate efficacy of interventions	Nursing staff	Chart/computer
Final design and development validation	Provide discharge instructions	Physician, social services, and/or nursing staff	Chart/computer, then to medical records.

The healthcare organization's design procedure should include details of how nursing care plan changes are identified, documented, and reviewed. The procedure should also establish who is authorized to review and approve design changes.

7.4 PURCHASING
7.4.1 PURCHASING PROCESS

A healthcare organization should maintain a process for conducting its purchasing activities. In many healthcare settings, especially hospitals, it is not uncommon to purchase all, or most, supplies from one source. A documented procedure would be helpful to establish the necessary purchasing controls. Points of interest for implementation include the necessity for determining whether all purchases are made by the same process. There may be many variations, and there may not be full knowledge at the administration level that managers or physicians are making independent purchases outside of the accepted process. Also, contracts for services, subcontract agreements, consulting arrangements, and so on, fall under this requirement.

The ANSI/ISO/ASQ Q9001-2000 standard requires that the healthcare organization evaluate, select, and reevaluate its suppliers. The term *supplier* is defined as an

IMPLEMENTATION GUIDANCE NOTE

A healthcare organization may elect to evaluate its vendors in a number of different ways.

Type of Evaluation	Evaluation Basis
Historical data	The basis for this selection method is normally based on past experience with the vendor/supplier. Current records will indicate whether the supplier has or has not provided goods or services on a consistent and reliable basis.
On-site assessment	This selection method is based on the healthcare organization's personnel visiting the vendor's/supplier's location and conducting a formal evaluation of its ability to provide acceptable products or services. On-site assessments may be conducted for: • Treatment programs purchased from suppliers • Verification and review of a vendor's/supplier's qualifications and facility • Audit of suppliers
Third-party registration	This selection method is based on the vendor/supplier maintaining a certified ISO 9001:2000 quality management system by an accredited independent certification body (registrar). The vendor's/supplier's certified quality management system should cover the products or services that the healthcare organization plans to purchase. A current copy of the vendor's/supplier's ISO 9001:2000 certificate should be on file.
Reputation	This selection method is based on the vendor's/supplier's reputation. References from other customers may also serve as objective evidence and serve as a means of such a selection.
Desktop evaluation	This selection method is based on a questionnaire sent to the vendors/suppliers asking them to self-evaluate their ability to provide acceptable products or services. The questionnaire is returned to the healthcare organization and evaluated for meeting specified criteria defined in the healthcare organization's documented procedure. If the review of the responses of the potential vendor/supplier is acceptable, they are then approved for use.
Provisional selection	This selection method is used when a new supplier is being considered on a trial basis over a specified period or for a specific application. Acceptance as a permanent supplier would depend on the results noted during the specified time period.

organization or individual that supplies or provides a product and/or service to the healthcare organization. Many healthcare providers use the term *vendor* instead of supplier. Healthcare providers may use the following chart for guidance when performing evaluations of vendors and suppliers.

There are many methods used to evaluate vendors/suppliers. Whatever the method or combination of methods used to assess suppliers, documented procedures should formulate the basis of assessing vendors/suppliers and potential vendors/suppliers.

ISO 9001:2000 requires a healthcare organization to define the type and extent of control that it will exercise over its vendors or subcontractors. For example, the control that the hospital has over physicians could be the peer review, credentialing and privileging process, or utilization review process. Studies are usually conducted at healthcare organizations to track unusual, costly, or repeated events such as high costs or high volume, problem prone, or high-risk areas. Through assessing such areas, the organization would be able to verify that their vendor/supplier evaluation and control process/system is implemented and that the vendors/suppliers have demonstrated their capability and performance.

7.4.2 PURCHASING INFORMATION

Requirements for purchasing information are typically met with ease: there must be a clear description of what was ordered. If there are requirements for approving the product, procedures to be used, processes, equipment, vendors/suppliers meeting certain qualifications, or vendors/suppliers needing a quality management system, these requirements must be clearly stated.

7.4.3 VERIFICATION OF PURCHASED PRODUCT

A healthcare organization's procedures should address receiving or incoming inspection and evaluation methods that are to be applied and what the acceptance criteria will be for incoming medical supplies and products. The purpose of receiving inspection is to ensure that the organization receives what it ordered. Additionally, such receiving activities can be used to evaluate the ongoing acceptability of vendors/suppliers to meet the healthcare provider's requirements. Incoming inspection or evaluations of supplies and products might also include inspecting new equipment, evaluating new services that are supplied, and materials to be used. In most healthcare organizations, receiving inspection usually consists of count, quantity, and inspection for damage.

7.5 PRODUCTION AND SERVICE PROVISION

This is the heart of the quality management system. The ISO 9001:2000 standard requires that the healthcare organization carry out its service delivery processes *under controlled conditions.* What does the word *control* imply? The ISO 9001:2000 standard uses the term *control* throughout; for example, *Control* of documents (Clause 4.2.3), *Control* of records (Clause 4.2.4), *Control* of nonconforming product (Clause 8.3), and so on, all have requirements for controlling the defined processes.

Control implies that activities and processes used to carry out the healthcare service delivery process must be managed, overseen, and organized in such a manner so as to provide customer confidence in the organization's ability to satisfy stated or implied needs.

Methods that a healthcare organization may employ to ensure effective control over its processes might include the following:

- Ensuring the availability of documentation or other reference information that the healthcare organization's personnel may require such as PDRs, care plans, radiographic position guides, and so on

- Ensuring that policies, protocols, process maps, flowcharts, work instructions, and other documents defining the methodology and processes are available for use by personnel

- Ensuring that adequate equipment needed to carry out the service delivery processes is available and in good working condition

- Ensuring that measuring and monitoring equipment is in a calibrated state and ready for use

Processes must be evaluated and defined. The healthcare organization should carefully study all delivery processes, both clinical and nonclinical, during the management system development phase of the implementation process. Such processes include:

- Outpatient services (nonsurgical)

- Outpatient services (surgery required)

- Emergency services (ambulatory)

- Emergency services (hospital admission required)

- Preadmission through discharge (nonsurgical)

- Preadmission through discharge (surgery required including ICU/CCU)

- Preadmission through discharge (obstetrics)

- Home health services

- Long-term care

- Skilled nursing

- Pathology and laboratory

- Blood bank

- Psychiatric services

- Physiotherapy services

- Reproductive health services

- Maintenance and facilities management department

- Social work services

- Open heart surgery facility

- Radiology or imaging services

Compliance with reference standards and codes is required by ISO 9001:2000. Due to the nature and number of regulatory requirements within the healthcare industry, it would be impossible to list all of these requirements. A list of applicable standards and codes should be available and under control at the healthcare facility. Such regulatory requirements may include HIPAA, OSHA, JCAHO, AOA, CAP, CLIA, state health department, or regulatory/certification regulations for a variety of individual services.

Continual improvement of the quality management system focuses on linking customer requirements (7.2.1 Determination of customer requirements related to the product) with both product/service characteristics (distinguishing features) and quality characteristics. ISO 9001:2000 Subclause 7.5.1(b) suggests that in order to effectively control service delivery, information that describes service delivery characteristics must be available throughout the organization.

ISO 9001:2000 Subclauses 4.1(a) and (b) state that the healthcare organization should identify the processes needed for the quality management system and their application throughout the organization as well as to determine the sequence and interactions of these processes. When considering how to address this requirement, most organizations utilize flowcharting or process maps of work processes.

Flowcharts or process maps are graphical representations of how a work process or activity is carried out. It describes the path or steps that a process follows from start to finish.

A process is a set of interrelated or interactive activities that transform inputs into outputs. Outputs from one process may become the inputs of another. For example, a patient presents at admissions for an elective surgery. The patient delivers the physician's order to admissions personnel. The physician's order (output document) becomes the input document that begins the admission process at the hospital. The resulting output created by the physician is the order. The input for the admissions personnel is the physician's order that was presented by the patient.

ISO 9001:2000 focuses on process management, continual improvement, and enhancing customer satisfaction. Effective process management mandates that core work processes be identified and improved upon. Continual improvement focuses on processes, and a process must be understood if improvement is to take place.

Figure 6.1 depicts a generic example of a flowchart or process map. A *parallelogram* depicts the process input (admissions receives the physician's order). *Rectangles*

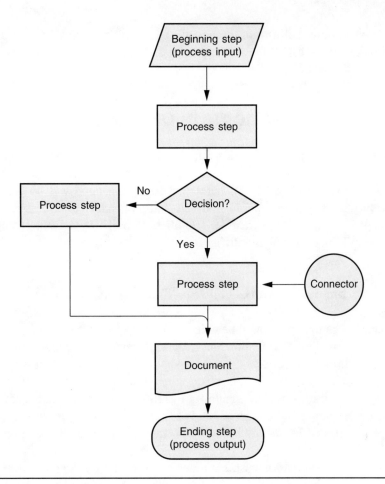

Figure 6.1   Basic flowcharting.

depict the process steps that will be carried out or executed (admissions reviews the physician's order). A *diamond* depicts when a decision must be made (Can the physician's requirements be met?). The *circle* indicates that there is a connection or interacting sequence between this process and another interrelated process or document (preadmission testing may have been required). The *rectangle* with *curved bottom* depicts that some document or record is to be referenced. This symbol may or may not be used (refer to the policy and procedure for admitting the patient and handling physician's orders).

The *rounded rectangle* completes the process and becomes the output from this process and the input for the next process (patient admitted, patient chart created, and chart and patient sent to floor).

Flowcharts may be basic and very linear in nature, or they may take more complex paths. A flowchart is a map, and a map provides directions from point *A* to point *B*. The process maps found in appendix C were used by the writer during several consultation projects. Flowcharts can illustrate the actual path a process takes and the ideal path a process should follow. ISO 9001:2000 internal audits (8.2.2 Internal audit) ensure that defined processes are being followed.

7.5.2 VALIDATION OF PROCESSES

Processes that may require validation include lab protocols, sterilization, radiology, mammography, pharmaceutical compounding, and so on. These processes must be validated and carried out by qualified personnel following approved procedures. Since healthcare providers would generally be using appropriately qualified personnel and established procedures for their treatment regimes, compliance with the requirements of this clause should not present any difficulties.

7.5.3 IDENTIFICATION AND TRACEABILITY

The healthcare organization should be able to identify and trace patients, relevant information, medical implants, correspondence, data, material, and other items throughout the facility. Additionally, patients/customers should be identified to ensure that appropriate treatment has been provided. For example, unique patient/customer identification systems can be used to provide traceability to relevant records. Banding of patients is one method. Bar coding and adhesive labels may also be used to provide identification and traceability of blood tests and blood by-products to associated documentation such as test records.

Data or records, such as assessment notes in medical records, may also be required under identification and traceability requirements. Subclause 4.2.4 Control of records covers the retention and storage of data and records, while 7.5.5 Preservation of product would be appropriate for materials.

7.5.4 CUSTOMER PROPERTY

The term *customer* may be defined as *the recipient of the service provided by the healthcare organization* (nonstaff doctors, patients, family members of patients, community at large, and so on); in contractual situations, the customer may also be referred to as the *patient*. The customer is the ultimate consumer, user, beneficiary, or purchaser of services provided by the healthcare organization. The customer may be internal or external to the organization.

Patient/customer property may be: personal belongings that the patient/customer provides to the healthcare facility, which may or may not be returned to the patient/customer. Examples of patient/customer property include patient-owned medications, banked blood or donated organs, and patient/customer clothing left in a locker room or patient room. Other examples include instruments used by physicians that are vendor

---

IMPLEMENTATION GUIDANCE NOTE

Here are some examples of where identification and traceability apply within the health-care organization.

Nursing	Pharmacy	Lab	Radiology	Food Services
Patient identification (bands, patient ID numbers)	Patient identification (bands, patient ID numbers)	Patient identification (bands, patient ID numbers)	Patient identification (bands, patient ID numbers)	Patient identification (bands, patient ID numbers)
Medical charts (Patient IDs)	Medication doses	Lab results, bar codes	Test results for scans and images	Food carts for delivery to floors
Treatment schedules	Controlled substances	Quality control/ test protocols	Treatment schedules	
Central sterile (ID of biological indicators)	Unit dose carts, medication sheets	Treatment schedules	Identification of radiographic sources	
Medical device (implantable) identification reporting and control	Identification and origin of medications			

---

samples or equipment that is not owned by the organization but supplied under some contractual arrangement.

A healthcare organization must ensure that all patient/customer property is identified, verified, stored, and maintained as required, using identification guidelines. If there are any problems with these items—becoming lost, damaged, or unuseable—the organization is required to report these conditions to the customer and keep a record. It should be noted that there is a relationship between Subclause 7.5.4 Customer property and 7.5.5 Preservation of product.

7.5.5 PRESERVATION OF PRODUCT

Preservation of product within the healthcare setting will be applied very broadly. Due to the types of services provided, preservation of product covers a wide range of areas and services throughout the healthcare infrastructure. This can include the safe transfer and mobility of patients from department to department, safe transportation of patients to and from the hospital, or medical records, x-rays, and test results supplied or provided by the patient. Handling patients and preserving products includes such items as tests, test specimens, and test reports for evaluation, medications, and/or other materials with a limited shelf life. Preservation also includes the protection of customer/patient possessions that the healthcare organization is responsible for or comes into contact with.

Limited shelf life is an important aspect to consider when documenting the ISO 9001:2000 preservation of product requirement. An example of the importance of verifying limited shelf life items was noted during the implementation of ISO 9001:2000 at an occupational health clinic. A container of long-expired *blind urine* was found in a refrigerator. Had the vial not been identified, this could have called into question all urine tests conducted by the clinic. Processes should be in place to ensure that stock is rotated and outdated supplies removed and destroyed. Many organizations use the *first in–first out* (FIFO) method of inventory rotation. Additionally, limited shelf life controls must be in place in the pharmacy, lab, food service areas, and so on, to ensure that the items in use are not expired.

Preservation of product also involves handling hazardous materials; checking MSDS sheets; and labeling and handling biohazards, reagents, and gases.

7.6 CONTROL OF MONITORING AND MEASURING DEVICES

Healthcare facilities maintain numerous measuring and monitoring devices. A procedure must be established to control the calibration process. Examples of where calibration may apply include:

- Equipment used for treatments where settings are critical such as defibrillators or gamma irradiation treatment equipment

- Diagnostic equipment

- Test equipment

- Software for which the need for calibration has been identified

- Measuring devices used in research projects

- Measuring devices, biological indicators used with autoclaves, freezers, and other equipment where pressure or temperature is critical

This clause sets requirements for identification and control of measurements to ensure that measuring and monitoring equipment, as well as equipment that could affect outcomes, or is used to verify outcomes, is appropriate for use, is properly maintained, and properly calibrated before use.

Calibration that is traceable to some national standard is not essential in all cases. For example, although surgical suite anesthetic gages need to be identified and calibrated, the gages on individual gas bottles connected via a manifold would only need a periodic check, provided that they are used to indicate an adequate supply (volume) of gas and not to measure pressure accurately during administration of gas to a patient. For some equipment, such as electronic equipment used to provide a go/no-go indication, periodic safety and function checks and maintenance may be adequate in lieu of calibration. Where there is a low risk of variation, some equipment may not require calibration at all. For example, thermometers, manometers, and cuffs may be exempt due to the low risk of variation relative to the application.

In addition to equipment, requirements for control may be needed. This control should include the accuracy of software applications where software operates assessment or test equipment and could affect patient outcomes.

Also, routine servicing and maintenance of measuring and test equipment would normally not satisfy the requirements for calibration (Clause 6.3 Infrastructure). In developing the procedures for calibration of measuring and monitoring devices, a healthcare organization should include the requirement that if a measuring or monitoring device is found to be outside of the calibration range, the consequences of possible inaccuracies of prior measurements need to be considered. If necessary, remedial action, such as recall or retesting, may need to be taken.

7

ISO 9001:2000 Clause 8— Measurement, Analysis and Improvement

Factual approach to decision making: the healthcare organization must base decisions on the logical or intuitive analysis of data and information.

8.1 GENERAL

Subclause 8.1 of ISO 9001:2000 deals with the third level of planning in the quality management system. The first level of planning was identified in Subclause 5.4 Planning. This planning is planning for the entire system and is conducted by top management or administration at the strategic level. The second level of planning within the ISO 9001:2000 standard is carried out in Clause 7.1 Planning of product realization and covers planning at the operational level. Here processes, service delivery, activities, and methods are planned and implemented with specifics and outcomes in mind. The third and final level of planning is found in Clause 8.1. The planning required in this section is conducted to identify and plan how the outcomes specified in level two are measured, monitored, and improved upon.

8.2.1 CUSTOMER SATISFACTION

Performance measures are already in use in nearly every healthcare setting. This requirement specifies that "information relating to customer perception as to whether the organization has met customer requirements" must be one of the ways to measure performance.

In healthcare settings, there may be some issues or problems in reconciling the differences between what a patient/customer may perceive as an acceptable healthcare outcome and what the healthcare provider can actually deliver by way of treatment, care plan, or care program. For example, a patient may *expect* that the healthcare provider can provide a *cure* for a particular health-related diagnosis, but the known medical knowledge on the condition can only provide a *management program* to control the symptoms. This scenario may play out even when the best possible service was delivered but the expectations were not achieved, thereby producing a negative perception of the outcome in the patient's mind. Handling such situations requires healthcare professionals to possess and demonstrate excellent communication skills. Determining customer perception of satisfaction involves a greater level of communication. Understanding what a customer feels is more subtle than hearing what the customer says, and is probably closer to the truth.

The process of delivering service in a healthcare setting is a very personal interaction, often with a patient and family in a state of crisis. It is important to manage a patient's perception of the quality of service being delivered during each and every interaction. It is possible to create a perception of quality service even though the patient may not be pleased during treatment and at the outcome of the episode of care. The perception of quality is created by interactions accomplished in a professional manner, by carefully communicating what the patient should expect, and by never failing to deliver agreed-upon activities in an accurate and timely fashion.

Healthcare organizations often rely on formal surveys to determine levels of service and patient satisfaction. These surveys are often conducted by third parties and take from three to 12 months to gather data, analyze the data, and formally report the information. While these surveys certainly add value to the knowledge base of the organization, they may have limited value for day-to-day operation because, by the time the report is received, the population surveyed received service from six to 12 months prior to the report.

Informal survey responses gathered at the point of service may have more value for the service provider who is concerned with managing specific customer perceptions on a continuous basis. The challenge is to formalize in a practical manner information that traditionally has been entirely verbal. Healthcare professionals rarely have an abundance of time, and one more requirement for record keeping can put them over the edge unless the method is relatively quick and painless.

8.2.2 INTERNAL AUDIT

Internal audit and reporting of opportunities for improvement is the cornerstone for continual improvement. This is one of the most essential aspects of ISO 9001:2000.

Healthcare organizations do not usually carry out self-assessment audits on all of the organization's activities, processes, and practices on a regular basis. The requirement for internal audits is usually an entirely new activity.

The ISO 9001:2000 standard requires that internal audits of the quality management system processes shall be carried out at defined intervals. Additionally, internal process/system audits shall cover evaluation of current practice to ensure that the requirements continue to be met.

Process/system audits (assessments) of the internal management structure are a relatively new concept in the healthcare community. Many healthcare organizations focus on *chart audits* and *compliance audits*. Neither of these audits are conducted to evaluate the service delivery system and processes throughout the entire healthcare organization but are narrowly focused in specific areas using specific audit criteria.

ISO 19011 is the audit standard published by the International Organization for Standardization. This document defines specific requirements for the qualification of audit personnel, defines audit methodology, and provides direction on managing the audit process. ISO 19011 is applicable to all organizations for carrying out both internal and external audits.

Audit Defined

ANSI/ISO/ASQ Q9000-2000 defines an internal audit as "a systematic, independent and documented process for obtaining audit evidence and evaluating it objectively to determine the extent to which audit criteria are fulfilled."

Elaborating on the definition, a *systematic* audit is one that is well planned and proceeds through the different stages of the audit lifecycle. It is *independent* in the sense that (per ANSI/ISO/ASQ Q9001-2000) "auditors shall not audit their own work." *Audit evidence* is defined as "records, statements of fact or other information which are relevant to the audit criteria and verifiable. Note: Audit evidence can be qualitative or quantitative." *Audit criteria* is defined as a "set of policies, procedures or requirements used as a reference."

Purpose of Auditing

There are several reasons for performing an audit of the quality system. The major reasons are:

1. To permit the listing of the audited organization's quality system in a register of certified organizations

2. To follow quality system standards, such as ISO 9001, that require internal audits

3. To meet regulatory requirements such as the Food and Drug Administration's Good Manufacturing Practices

4. To assist with the selection of suppliers

5. To determine the conformity or nonconformity of the quality system elements with specified requirements such as ISO 9001:2000

6. To assure management requirements that the quality system can deliver services that meet agreed patient/customer requirements and expectations

7. To determine the effectiveness of the implemented quality system in meeting specified quality objectives

Continuous improvement rather than compliance may be the major issue as a management system matures. The audit is used as a proactive tool to identify opportunities for improvement throughout the system.

A number of ISO 9001:2000 subclauses are closely associated with improvement. These include Internal audit (Subclause 8.2.2), Continual improvement (Subclause 8.5.1), Corrective action (Subclause 8.5.2), Preventive action (Subclause 8.5.3), and Management review (Subclause 5.6).

The Auditor's Responsibilities

Auditors are responsible for:

- Complying with the applicable audit requirements

- Communicating and clarifying audit requirements

- Planning and carrying out assigned responsibilities effectively and efficiently

- Documenting observations

- Reporting audit results

- Verifying the effectiveness of corrective actions taken as a result of the audit

- Retaining and safeguarding documents pertaining to the audit and submitting any required documents

- Ensuring that documents remains confidential

- Treating privileged information with discretion

Human Aspects of Conducting Internal Audits

The initial attempt at implementing an audit system often meets resistance of varying degrees in most organizations. There is natural resistance to any change, but people especially do not like change forced upon them. The greater the extent to which the change is being done *to* them rather than *by* them, the greater the resistance to the change. Implementing ISO 9001:2000 within a healthcare setting is often very difficult due to the resistance that staff have to change. There may be a long history of *we've always done it this way* to overcome.

In the case of implementing an internal auditing activity, the cultural change that people will experience is sometimes both intrusive and critical—not only will their work areas be invaded but their work efforts may also be critiqued. People who have been performing their jobs, perhaps for years, without scrutiny will now have their behavior subjected to the review of others.

For this reason, the auditing function should not be justified based on some external need for its existence. It does not comfort a fearful staff or other healthcare professionals to know that the auditing system is required by standards such as ISO 9001:2000. They really do not care!

The reason that ISO 9001:2000 requires internal auditing is because it has intrinsic organizational value. Staff and other healthcare professionals will be more receptive to auditing if they know that its purpose is to find the causes of job-related problems, so that those problems may be eliminated and hopefully make their jobs easier. This is a cultural issue; if the healthcare provider is introducing auditing into the workplace, the audit manager or management representative must become the change agent. The auditing function will operate smoothly if it is accepted as a valuable improvement tool. Therefore, much of the work in setting up an internal auditing process in the healthcare organization is devoted to gaining acceptance for its value.

To gain acceptance, the audit manager or management representative must educate the work force. Education can be handled through newsletters, memos, e-mail, departmental meetings, and other available means. It is essential that the workforce get answers to these questions about auditing:

- What is an audit?

- How is it conducted?

- Why is it done?

- What are the benefits to the healthcare organization?

- What are the benefits to the staff and other healthcare professionals?

- Why should staff not fear an audit?

One tactic that some healthcare organizations have used when implementing an internal audit system is to *first tell them and then show them.* In this approach, everyone is first informed about how auditing can be a benefit to people in their own work space. Then, pilot or mentored audits are conducted. The results are reported along with whatever problems were found, and subsequent corrective actions (opportunities for improvement) are identified. When people see that the audit works to their benefit the way they were told it would, they begin to overcome their fears.

If a healthcare organization is going to make the audit process work, auditors and potential auditors must be carefully selected and instructed. Ideally, auditors should be good at putting people at ease and remaining focused on issues that will help a department improve. Typically, administrator- and director-level personnel should not conduct audits. Also, the organization will not want auditors who are arrogant or nitpickers.

Management must be prepared if the audit process is going to work. Quality system auditing, like other quality related functions, should be described to management in terms of how it helps the healthcare organization achieve its business and strategic goals, targets, and objectives. If auditing is perceived to be something apart from the business of the healthcare organization, it will not be afforded much attention. If it is understood to be a tool to help uncover and remove problems that prevent the healthcare organization from operating effectively, economically, and efficiently, then it will be valued. Once management understands this, they will be open to using the tool properly.

If individual contributors in the healthcare organization are to accept the value of the auditing process, management must first accept it.

Managers do not want to be judged by the number of problems found in their areas—especially if they have become successful by covering up problems. If they think they will be judged in this manner, they may shift the blame for problems to individual employees, doing exactly what the audit manager or management representative said would not be done. Management must be convinced that auditing is a beneficial tool, not a harmful weapon.

The Internal Audit Procedure

After obtaining management commitment, the next step is to define the audit infrastructure, describe the audit process, and write a detailed audit procedure, so that audit consistency can be achieved. The audit procedure details responsibilities and activities of the audit management, audit coordinator, audit team leader, audit team, auditee, and management. The procedure thoroughly defines the audit process and typically includes planning and execution of the audit, reporting results, documenting the audit, follow-up of corrective action, closeout of the audit, and record retention. The procedure is all-inclusive and leaves no requirement unstated.

One important feature that should be included in any internal audit procedure is the process that describes the avenue of escalation for issues that cannot be resolved at the manager level. These issues might include delaying tactics by the auditee in scheduling an audit, disputed audit findings that cannot be resolved by the parties involved, or lack of response from the auditee in submitting a corrective action plan to the audit manager. Having a defined escalation process in place can remove the emotions involved in cases of disagreement or dispute.

8.2.3 AND 8.2.4 MONITORING AND MEASUREMENT OF PROCESSES AND PRODUCT

The standard requires monitoring of both process and product. A problem for the healthcare provider may be understanding what a process is and what a product is. When the product is service delivery, the distinction is not always entirely clear. Simply put, monitoring the process is ensuring that activities described in procedures are performed the way the procedure describes and determining the efficiency with which procedures are carried out. Monitoring the product is monitoring the outcome of procedures.

The healthcare organization needs to establish appropriate assessments, tests, or verifications to be performed at the various stages of the healthcare delivery process. The assessments, tests, or verifications should be consistent with the service delivery, methods, and operations and should be defined in appropriate procedures.

For example, measuring and monitoring (assessment and inspection) may be applied to incoming patients with respect to the recognition of prior treatment and medical history, assessment of patients and development of treatment and care plans at admission, check of progress against the original interventions defined for each stage of the patient's care plan, and identification of special considerations or possible difficulties for a particular patient. These same considerations could also be addressed under ISO 9001:2000 Subclause 7.2.2 Review of requirements related to the product.

In many cases, policies and procedures will cover the process and any assessment, testing, or verification requirements. For example, assessment of patient/customer treatment or care plans could be addressed under this clause or Subclause 7.5. These two clauses cover the monitoring and measuring of processes and service delivery. In many instances, the same techniques will apply to both. For example, measuring how successful a treatment regime has been will, of necessity, measure the outcome of the delivered service with respect to the patient's status. Monitoring and measuring could also apply to:

- Assessing and evaluating patient/customer outcomes

- Monitoring treatment programs such as a rehabilitation program

- Monitoring administration systems

- Ensuring that equipment is functioning correctly

- Checking the continuing suitability of equipment and facilities

- Monitoring the use of consumable items such as wheelchairs or food

8.3 CONTROL OF NONCONFORMING PRODUCT

In healthcare organizations, a nonconformity is often known as a variance, occurrence, or incident and is reported as such. Some examples of nonconformities in the healthcare facility include:

- The inability to admit patients due to waiting lists or unavailability of beds

- Inadequate or inappropriate materials and services provided by the healthcare organization

- Equipment that is not functioning correctly, is out of service, or is out of calibration

- Out-of-date food, medication, or drugs that has not been disposed of properly

- The failure to meet legislative or regulatory requirements

- The failure to follow or meet procedures, standards, or organizational guidelines

- Deficiencies in the quality management system or procedures

- Patient falls

The following situation shows when a nonconformity becomes reportable. A laboratory technician or pharmacist prepares incorrect materials or formulary for a test procedure or medication. The technician then discovers and rectifies the error before the test is started, or before the medication leaves the pharmacy, and the error is corrected. So far, this does not constitute a nonconformance. However, if the medical director or director of pharmacy discovers the error during a check of the test or medication, or the nonconforming medication leaves the pharmacy and is later discovered, this is a nonconformance that must be reported and corrective action taken to determine whether lab or pharmacy processes are effective or need improvement to preclude recurrence.

8.4 ANALYSIS OF DATA

ISO requires an organization to "determine, collect and analyze appropriate data to demonstrate the suitability and effectiveness of the quality management system." The challenge for healthcare is not to have data but to keep appropriate data for a specific reason. Too often, data is collected by managers who do not know whether the data has a real and vital function in the organization or not. It is just something they are required to do. And all too often there is no real value. Some reports exist for the sole reason that a manager who is no longer with the organization set them up once upon a time. The routine has continued long after its value disappeared.

Healthcare organizations typically collect reams of clinical data with little if any data collected for nonclinical areas. Support services are critical to the ongoing effectiveness of healthcare delivery processes, and data needs to be analyzed and evaluated for these critical areas. The healthcare organization must collect information and manage it in a way that supports the healthcare organization's strategic and operational plans and objectives.

Areas where analysis (including statistical techniques) might apply include:

- Patient/customer satisfaction analysis

- Preventive action

- Collection and analysis of process information

- Performance of suppliers

Patient/customer data and clinical information should be analyzed to provide comparative analysis of outcomes, occurrences, incidents, and variances and to provide information that can become the basis for continual quality improvement (CQI). Where data is used to compare performance and evaluate outcomes, it is important that the procedures for collecting, reporting, and exchanging information are compatible and based on sound statistical methods.

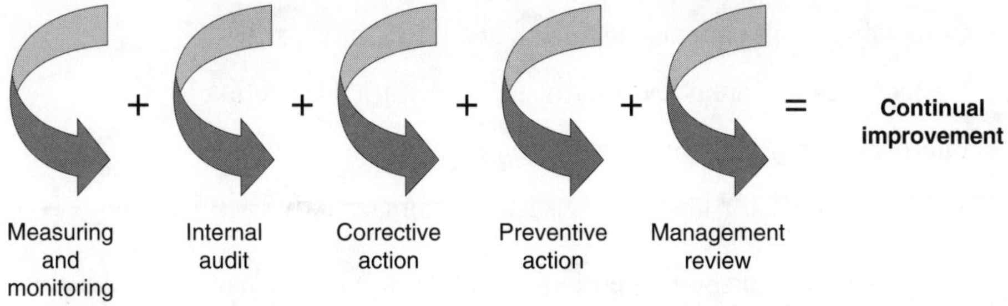

Figure 7.1 Five keys to continual improvement.

8.5.1 CONTINUAL IMPROVEMENT

A healthcare organization needs to have a plan on how the quality management system can be improved. This organizational improvement is known as *continual improvement,* a familiar term to healthcare organizations. The five keys to continual improvement of an ISO 9001:2000 quality management system are depicted in Figure 7.1. When implementing an ISO 9001:2000 quality management system, the measuring and monitoring of both processes and service delivery must ensure that effective controls have been applied to the process and that healthcare service is being delivered in accordance with planned arrangements.

Improvement has long been a goal or objective in healthcare; most organizations have a performance improvement component in their organizational structure, yet real, sustained improvement is often elusive. The ISO standard not only requires improvement but indicates how the improvement is to be obtained: by using quality objectives, audit results, analysis of data, corrective actions, preventive actions, and management review. When these components of the quality management system are implemented with care, the expected outcome is improvement. Improvement becomes a predictable result rather than an elusive hope.

8.5.2 CORRECTIVE ACTION

Both corrective and preventive actions are activities and steps in the quality and organizationwide improvement cycle. Corrective action is initiated by the occurrence of a nonconformity, patient/customer complaint, or similar event. Corrective action is taken to ensure that the cause of a problem is identified and action is taken to prevent recurrence of the problem.

The requirement for corrective action is one of the six ISO clauses that specifically require a procedure. An effective procedure would ensure constant and consistent review of:

- Adverse events and outcomes relating to patient/customer care

- Nonconformities, variances, occurrences, and incidents

- Complaints from patients/customers and other third parties

- Deficiencies and areas for improvement identified by audits

- Internal reports, including suggestions

These reviews are for the purpose of initiating corrective action when it is appropriate to do so.

The points reviewed should be monitored by top management or administration as key elements of an integrated system of incident, variances, occurrences, and nonconformity reporting, and continual quality improvement. Investigative and root cause analysis tools should be used to identify contributing factors and enable corrective actions to be taken. The healthcare organization should also identify the cause of any problems arising from any failure of the quality management system, complaints from suppliers, or unsatisfactory procedures.

Irrespective of how the need for corrective action is identified, the healthcare organization should ensure that appropriate action is initiated and corrective action taken. Top management and administration should ensure that the changes resulting from corrective action are followed up on to make sure that they are effective.

8.5.3 PREVENTIVE ACTION

Preventive action is concerned with analyzing the system using the available data and other appropriate information to identify causes of potential problems before problems occur, thus eliminating possible causes of nonconformity or patient/customer complaints. This proactive approach built into the quality management system is an opportunity to base quality improvements on good ideas alone. Too many companies do nothing more than solve problems as they arise; while it is necessary to solve problems, this approach tends to eat up any and all available energy, leaving little opportunity for other activities.

The path for preventive action, once the action has been identified, is the same as the ISO requirements for corrective action. Take appropriate action, record the results, and then review the action taken to see if it was effective.

8

Conclusion

PUTTING ALL THE PIECES TOGETHER

The previous chapters have discussed the philosophy of the ISO standard and have defined the requirements specified in ISO 9001:2000. Implementation guidance notes have provided healthcare organizations with a road map for implementing the standard. Once the organization has decided to implement ISO 9001:2000, there are several decisions that must be made before the real work can begin.

First, the organization should decide whether a change agent or consultant is necessary to assist. Typically, a change agent or consultant is an outside independent firm that has no preconceived notions about the internal workings of the organization, and that can assist in facilitating effective implementation of the standard. The healthcare provider should choose this consultant carefully. Select only those consulting firms that are themselves ISO 9001:2000 certified and have a proven track record of implementing ISO 9000 within other healthcare organizations. A consulting firm that is ISO 9001:2000 certified demonstrates to the healthcare organization that there are defined and documented processes and methods for measuring customer satisfaction in the firm's system and that the firm has its own continual quality improvement initiative. Ask the firm for copies of its ISO 9001:2000 certificate and copies of satisfaction surveys or records that demonstrate service delivery performance. Beware of consulting firms that are not ISO 9001:2000 registered. Such noncertified/nonregistered consulting firms have made a conscious decision to not document their processes and practices nor to improve upon what they do. They have not implemented ISO 9001:2000 for a reason.

If a healthcare provider elects to implement ISO 9001:2000 themselves without assistance from a consulting firm, the first step is to establish an ISO team or committee. Using this book as an implementation guide, create a project plan and begin writing procedures and drafting work flows and processes.

At some point in the project, the healthcare organization should have internal auditor training. Choose a Registrar Accreditation Board (RAB) accredited internal auditor course provider to conduct an internal auditor training course so that there is confidence that the training meets all requirements of the RAB. Please visit the RAB list of approved course providers at:

http://www.rabnet.com/rab/searchCP.do?currentCourseType=5&currentState=ALL&currentCountry=-1&currentSector=-1.

When all requirements of ISO 9001:2000 have been documented and implemented, the final step for certification is to select a registrar to perform the certification audit. There is a list of accredited registrars on the same Web site: www.rabnet.com. Be sure to verify that the registrar is qualified in the healthcare industry. Registrars must have the appropriate industry in their scope of accreditation before they can provide an organization with an accredited certificate.

In conclusion, embarking on the journey toward excellence and continual improvement begins with understanding and applying the ISO 9001:2000 standard. It is the standard for quality worldwide. It is the American standard for quality. It is the standard that will change the face of healthcare quality.

A recent study conducted by the University of Maryland, R. H. Smith School of Business, the Anderson School at UCLA, and the Universidad Carlos III in Madrid, Spain, indicated that U.S. publicly held companies trading on the New York Stock Exchange that were certified to the ISO 9000 quality management standards showed significant improvement in financial performance compared to companies that had not implemented the standard. The study's findings also included the following:

- Organizations that failed to seek certification experienced substantial deterioration in return on assets, productivity, and sales while certified companies avoided such declines.

- Organizations that received certification had improved performance compared to their peers that were not ISO 9000 certified.

- Chemical companies, in the two years prior to certification, showed a relative difference in return on assets between certified and uncertified organizations of less than five percent; three years after certification the difference was 12 percent.

- Organizations, immediately after deciding to seek certification, experienced a productivity improvement while noncertified organizations saw no such improvement and, in fact, eventually experienced a gradual decline.

The question for healthcare providers is not, "Should we comply with ISO 9001:2000?" Rather, the question is, "Can we afford not to comply with ISO 9001:2000?"

Appendix A

ISO 9001:2000
Self-Assessment Tool

ISO 9001:2000 is an international standard that defines requirements to assist health-care organizations in building a system for managing the systems and processes within their facilities.

The standard specifies requirements that must be met for a quality management system. Your application of the standard should reflect the mission and values of your organization; beginning with a succinct quality policy statement and set objectives, all facets of the quality management system focus on those goals and drive them to reality.

SCORING THE SELF-ASSESSMENT INSTRUMENT

Perspective

Take the perspective of people who do the daily work within the healthcare organization rather than what management wants or leadership says. In other words, be as objective as possible about the reality of your current systems and processes.

Scoring

Respond to each statement with a percentage of readiness corresponding to one of the following phrases that best describes how well your organization performs with respect to that statement.

For statements related to *documentation* (prefixed by a *D* on the score sheets), use these phrases:

> 20 percent—There has been discussion about the need for documentation.
>   (Or do not know.)

40 percent—Rough drafts or outdated versions exist but are not used.

60 percent—Documentation exists, but it is superficial, is seen as insufficient, or not useful.

80 percent—Documentation exists and is generally useful, but it is not always kept up-to-date.

100 percent—Relevant documentation is available, complete, useful, and up-to-date.

For statements related to *implementation* (prefixed by an *I* on the score sheets), use these phrases:

20 percent—There has been discussion about the need for this. (Or do not know.)

40 percent—Applies to limited parts of the organization.

60 percent—Widespread awareness exists, but not done on a consistent basis across the organization.

80 percent—Consistently done in major parts of the organization, and done sporadically in other parts.

100 percent—The norm for all major parts of the organization.

For the purpose of this tool, the ISO 9001:2000 standard has been broken into three parts: Leadership and Quality Improvement, Quality System Infrastructure, and Process Management in Quality Organizations. At the end of each section you will find score sheets, which are self-explanatory. The last page of the tool is a final scoring sheet. Tally up the results from the section score sheets and place them in the appropriate columns. Divide the total number by 20 and you will have your organizational percentage of readiness to obtain ISO 9001:2000 certification.

Note: In some cases, all of the questions will not apply to your organization. If this is the case, simply add the scores that you did answer in a specific section and divide that number by the total number of questions answered. We hope that you find this tool useful as you consider adding ISO 9001 to your current management system in order to bring about continuous quality improvement.

Leadership and Quality Improvement

5 Management responsibility 5.3 Quality policy	Documentation	Implementation
LD1. A written quality policy (mission, vision statement) authorized by top management is published and maintained. Additionally, specific objectives, goals, and targets have been developed and are available to staff.	☐ ☐ ☐ ☐ ☐ 20 40 60 80 100	
LD2. Copies of the quality policy (mission, vision statement) and objectives are available to employees.	☐ ☐ ☐ ☐ ☐ 20 40 60 80 100	
LD3. Employees can restate the intent of the quality policy (mission, vision statement) and describe how it applies to them.		☐ ☐ ☐ ☐ ☐ 20 40 60 80 100
LD4. Procedures exist to ensure that new employees are oriented to the quality policy (mission, vision statement).	☐ ☐ ☐ ☐ ☐ 20 40 60 80 100	
LD5. Organizational strategies as well as quality concerns are reviewed and addressed using the quality policy (mission, vision statement) as the basis for making decisions.		☐ ☐ ☐ ☐ ☐ 20 40 60 80 100
5 Management responsibility 5.5.1 Responsibility and authority		
LD6. Responsibilities and authorities for all personnel are clearly defined and documented.	☐ ☐ ☐ ☐ ☐ 20 40 60 80 100	
LD7. All personnel have written job descriptions with responsibility and authority clearly specified.	☐ ☐ ☐ ☐ ☐ 20 40 60 80 100	
LD8. There is a current documented and approved organizational chart in place.	☐ ☐ ☐ ☐ ☐ 20 40 60 80 100	
LD9. Authority is delegated to appropriate personnel to identify and record service delivery deficiencies (nonconformity). These personnel have the authority to initiate and verify corrective action and control further activities.		☐ ☐ ☐ ☐ ☐ 20 40 60 80 100
LD10. Specific authority is delegated to identify and record service delivery deficiencies (nonconformity, occurrence, variances).		☐ ☐ ☐ ☐ ☐ 20 40 60 80 100
LD11. Specific authority is assigned for review of service delivery deficiencies (nonconformity, occurrence, variances) to determine what corrective and/or preventive action is necessary.		☐ ☐ ☐ ☐ ☐ 20 40 60 80 100
LD12. Specific authority for initiating solutions to service delivery deficiencies (nonconformity, occurrence, variances) through designated channels is documented.		☐ ☐ ☐ ☐ ☐ 20 40 60 80 100

Leadership and Quality Improvement

5 Management responsibility 5.5.2 Management representative	Documentation	Implementation
LD17. There is a written document defining the appointment of a management representative.	☐ ☐ ☐ ☐ ☐ 20 40 60 80 100	
LD18. The designated management representative is active, visible, credible, and effective. This person ensures that the requirements of ISO 9001:2000 are established, implemented, and maintained and reports to top management on management system performance.		☐ ☐ ☐ ☐ ☐ 20 40 60 80 100
5 Management responsibility **5.6 Management review**		
LD19. The quality manual describes methods for conducting formal management reviews of the quality system effectiveness: frequency and scope of reviews, who participates, how recommendations are acted upon, how results are tracked, and how minutes are kept.	☐ ☐ ☐ ☐ ☐ 20 40 60 80 100	
LD20. Management review has been carried out in order to verify the continuing effectiveness of the quality management system.		☐ ☐ ☐ ☐ ☐ 20 40 60 80 100
LD21. Records or minutes of management reviews (outputs) indicate that procedures have been followed, recommendations made, actions taken, and changes to the quality system are implemented.	☐ ☐ ☐ ☐ ☐ 20 40 60 80 100	
4 Quality management system **4.2.1 General and 4.2.2 Quality manual**		
QI1. A documented quality systems manual assures that stated policies and objectives for service quality performance have been established in accordance with ISO 9001:2000. The manual is sufficiently specific to guide personnel on *who, where,* and *why.*	☐ ☐ ☐ ☐ ☐ 20 40 60 80 100	
QI2. A quality systems manual is implemented and describes the organization's procedural infrastructure which acts as a road map to guide and navigate users to the applicable quality system procedures and protocols that drive organizationwide quality and performance.		☐ ☐ ☐ ☐ ☐ 20 40 60 80 100
QI3. The quality system documentation is easily understood by all personnel who have a need to use it.	☐ ☐ ☐ ☐ ☐ 20 40 60 80 100	
QI4. There are written plans of care, clinical pathways, nursing plans, PI plans (how the requirements for quality will be met) for each patient, service delivery activity, or project engaged in.		☐ ☐ ☐ ☐ ☐ 20 40 60 80 100
QI5. Personnel use, carry out, and follow the plans of care, clinical pathways, nursing plans, and PI plans (how the requirements for quality will be met) to ensure that quality objectives and clinical outcome expectations are met.		☐ ☐ ☐ ☐ ☐ 20 40 60 80 100

Leadership and Quality Improvement

4 Quality management system 4.2.1 General and 4.2.2 Quality manual	Documentation	Implementation
QI6. Personnel throughout the organization are aware of policies, procedures, protocols, and instructions, and know where to get them.		☐ ☐ ☐ ☐ ☐ 20 40 60 80 100
QI7. Personnel understand policies, procedures, protocols, and instructions and use them to ensure acceptable and consistent service delivery as well as to obtain measurable outcomes.		☐ ☐ ☐ ☐ ☐ 20 40 60 80 100
8 Measurement, analysis and improvement 8.2.2 Internal audit		
QI8. Written procedures address how to plan, schedule, document, and follow up on internal quality audits of the entire quality system.	☐ ☐ ☐ ☐ ☐ 20 40 60 80 100	
QI9. Internal audit personnel have been trained and audits are conducted at defined intervals. Improvements to the system are recommended and action is taken. If necessary, changes to the quality system are made and their effectiveness is verified.		☐ ☐ ☐ ☐ ☐ 20 40 60 80 100
QI10. The results of all internal audits are documented and reported to management.	☐ ☐ ☐ ☐ ☐ 20 40 60 80 100	
QI11. Management reviews the results of the internal quality audits during its annual management review and makes a determination as to the continuing suitability and effectiveness of the documented quality system in order to continue meeting patient/customer needs and expectations.		☐ ☐ ☐ ☐ ☐ 20 40 60 80 100
8 Measurement, analysis and improvement 8.5.2 Corrective action		
QI12. Procedures exist for implementing corrective actions to eliminate the *causes* of nonconforming service delivery and/or poor patient care and inefficient processes.	☐ ☐ ☐ ☐ ☐ 20 40 60 80 100	
QI13. Procedures exist that define the effective handling of customer/patient complaints, investigate the *causes* of such complaints, determine the corrective actions needed to eliminate the *causes* of customer/patient complaints, and define controls necessary to ensure that corrective action is effective.	☐ ☐ ☐ ☐ ☐ 20 40 60 80 100	
QI14. Corrective action procedures not only deal effectively with problems in the present and near term, but records indicate that the procedures have been useful in driving continuous quality improvement.		☐ ☐ ☐ ☐ ☐ 20 40 60 80 100
QI15. Records indicate that corrective action has been brought to management's attention for use during management review to evaluate the continued suitability and effectiveness of the management system.		☐ ☐ ☐ ☐ ☐ 20 40 60 80 100

Leadership and Quality Improvement

8 Measurement, analysis and improvement 8.5.3 Preventive action	Documentation	Implementation
QI16. Procedures exist for implementing preventive actions to eliminate the *potential causes* of nonconforming service delivery and/or poor patient care.	☐ ☐ ☐ ☐ ☐ 20 40 60 80 100	
QI17. Procedures define what sources of organizational data and other outcome measures will be used to detect, analyze, and eliminate *potential causes* of nonconforming service delivery and/or poor patient care.	☐ ☐ ☐ ☐ ☐ 20 40 60 80 100	
QI18. Records indicate that appropriate steps are taken to deal effectively with *potential* problems requiring preventive action.		☐ ☐ ☐ ☐ ☐ 20 40 60 80 100
QI19. Personnel initiate preventive action and ensure that the preventive measures taken are effective.		☐ ☐ ☐ ☐ ☐ 20 40 60 80 100
QI20. Records indicate that preventive actions have been brought to management's attention for use during the annual evaluation of the effectiveness of the overall quality system.		☐ ☐ ☐ ☐ ☐ 20 40 60 80 100
4 Quality management system **4.2.4 Control of records**		
QI21. Procedures exist to guide the organization in identifying, collecting, filing, indexing, storing, maintaining, retaining, and disposing of records (clinical and nonclinical).	☐ ☐ ☐ ☐ ☐ 20 40 60 80 100	
QI22. Procedures outline how records are held in confidence and are stored to minimize deterioration and allow for easy retrieval.	☐ ☐ ☐ ☐ ☐ 20 40 60 80 100	
QI23. The quality records system works well and facilitates information retrieval for root cause analysis whether initiated by patient/customer complaints or process control difficulties.		☐ ☐ ☐ ☐ ☐ 20 40 60 80 100
8 Measurement, analysis and improvement **8.4 Analysis of data**		
QI24. Procedures exist for the application of statistical techniques to control and measure service delivery processes, collect data for measurable clinical outcomes, and assist in identifying problems involving poor organizational performance.	☐ ☐ ☐ ☐ ☐ 20 40 60 80 100	
QI25. Procedures exist for the application of statistical techniques to control and measure service delivery processes, collect data for measurable clinical outcomes, and assist in identifying problems involving poor organizational performance.		☐ ☐ ☐ ☐ ☐ 20 40 60 80 100
QI26. Pareto charts and/or other statistical techniques are used to identify and track quality/service delivery problems in order to identify root causes of those problems and report the same to management.	☐ ☐ ☐ ☐ ☐ 20 40 60 80 100	

Leadership and Quality Improvement

Section Scoring Sheet 1	Documentation	Implementation
5 Management responsibility *D* Score + *I* Score = [ ] Total Section Score Divide the section score by 17 = [ ] Section Average Score	LD1 _____ LD2 _____ LD4 _____ LD6 _____ LD7 _____ LD8 _____ LD17 _____ LD19 _____ LD21 _____ *D* Score _____	LD3 _____ LD5 _____ LD9 _____ LD10 _____ LD11 _____ LD12 _____ LD18 _____ LD20 _____ *I* Score _____
4 Quality management system *D* Score + *I* Score = [ ] Total Section Score Divide the section score by 7 = [ ] Section Average Score	QI1 _____ QI3 _____ QI4 _____ *D* Score _____	QI2 _____ QI5 _____ QI6 _____ QI7 _____ *I* Score _____
8.2.2 Internal audit *D* Score + *I* Score = [ ] Total Section Score Divide the section score by 4 = [ ] Section Average Score	QI8 _____ QI10 _____ *D* Score _____	QI9 _____ QI11 _____ *I* Score _____
8.5.2 Corrective action **8.5.3 Preventive action** *D* Score + *I* Score = [ ] Total Section Score Divide the section score by 9 = [ ] Section Average Score	QI12 _____ QI13 _____ QI16 _____ QI17 _____ *D* Score _____	QI14 _____ QI15 _____ QI18 _____ QI19 _____ QI20 _____ *I* Score _____

Leadership and Quality Improvement

Section Scoring Sheet 1	Documentation	Implementation

4.2.4 Control of records
 	
D Score + *I* Score = ☐
      Total Section
      Score
 	
Divide the section = ☐
  score by 3
      Section
      Average
      Score
	QI21 _____
	QI22 _____
	
	D Score _____
		QI23 _____
		
		I Score _____

8.4 Analysis of data
 	
D Score + *I* Score = ☐
      Total Section
      Score
 	
Divide the section = ☐
  score by 3
      Section
      Average
      Score
	QI24 _____
	QI26 _____
	
	D Score _____
		QI25 _____
		
		I Score _____

Quality System Infrastructure

4 Quality management system 4.2.3 Control of documents	Documentation	Implementation
TX1. Procedures describe a control mechanism that ensures that all documents (policies, procedures, protocols, instructions, forms) are controlled.	☐ ☐ ☐ ☐ ☐ 20 40 60 80 100	
TX2. Procedures, protocols, instructions, and forms are approved by authorized personnel prior to issue.	☐ ☐ ☐ ☐ ☐ 20 40 60 80 100	
TX3. Documents of external origin such as accreditation standards, FDA, DEA, state HD regulations, or HCFA are controlled to ensure that the latest versions or revisions are available to personnel who need the documents.		☐ ☐ ☐ ☐ ☐ 20 40 60 80 100
TX4. Current revisions of policies, procedures, protocols, instructions, and forms are readily available and in use by all personnel.		☐ ☐ ☐ ☐ ☐ 20 40 60 80 100
TX5. A master list of documents identifying the current revision status of policies, procedures, protocols, instructions, and forms is available to preclude the use of invalid and/or obsolete documents.	☐ ☐ ☐ ☐ ☐ 20 40 60 80 100	
TX6. Invalid and/or obsolete policies, procedures, protocols, instructions, and forms are promptly removed from all points of use and replaced with updated revisions.		☐ ☐ ☐ ☐ ☐ 20 40 60 80 100
TX7. Obsolete policies, procedures, protocols, instructions, and forms retained for knowledge preservation purposes are suitably identified.		☐ ☐ ☐ ☐ ☐ 20 40 60 80 100
TX8. Changes and revisions to policies, procedures, protocols, instructions, and forms are reviewed and approved by the same *function* as those who performed the original review and approval.		☐ ☐ ☐ ☐ ☐ 20 40 60 80 100
TX9. Procedures describe a method for safeguarding computer data. Appropriate backup procedures exist. Computer process management control software systems such as Meditech are safeguarded and protected to ensure confidentiality.	☐ ☐ ☐ ☐ ☐ 20 40 60 80 100	
TX10. Records indicate that computer backups occur on a regular basis. Backups are safeguarded.		☐ ☐ ☐ ☐ ☐ 20 40 60 80 100
7 Product realization **7.5.4 Customer property**		
TX11. Procedures for verification, storage, identification, recording, and maintaining patient valuables and other personal effects, which the organization will be required to control while the patient is under the organization's control, exist.	☐ ☐ ☐ ☐ ☐ 20 40 60 80 100	
TX12. Personnel understand the protocols for the control of patient-owned items. Items are rarely lost, damaged, or misused.		☐ ☐ ☐ ☐ ☐ 20 40 60 80 100

Quality System Infrastructure

7 Product realization 7.5.3 Identification and traceability (Patient Identification Protocols/Medical Product Traceability)	Documentation	Implementation
TX13. Organizationwide procedures and protocols describe the process of identifying critical medical products (pharmaceuticals, blood, medical devices, etc.) purchased by the hospital and used in providing patient care.	❏ ❏ ❏ ❏ ❏ 20 40 60 80 100	
TX14. Procedures and/or protocols exist describing the process of identifying patients throughout the healthcare delivery process.	❏ ❏ ❏ ❏ ❏ 20 40 60 80 100	
TX15. Identification and traceability records indicate a high degree of traceability and identification controls. Such records are available in a timely manner.		❏ ❏ ❏ ❏ ❏ 20 40 60 80 100
TX16. Critical medical products (meds, blood, medical devices, etc.) are identified in such a manner that positive recall of such products can be accomplished easily.		❏ ❏ ❏ ❏ ❏ 20 40 60 80 100
7.5.3 Identification and traceability (Assessment, Examination and Test Status)		
TX17. Procedures and protocols exist that describe the assessment or examination status of the patient or their tests.	❏ ❏ ❏ ❏ ❏ 20 40 60 80 100	
TX18. Assessment, examination, and test status procedures or protocols work well. There are no known instances of assessments or tests that were not conducted as ordered. Little time is wasted because of confusion over test results.		❏ ❏ ❏ ❏ ❏ 20 40 60 80 100
8 Measurement, analysis and improvement **8.3 Control of nonconforming product** (Control of Nonconforming Service)		
TX19. Procedures exist to ensure that medical supplies that do not conform to specified requirements are prevented from inadvertent use.	❏ ❏ ❏ ❏ ❏ 20 40 60 80 100	
TX20. Procedures exist to ensure that service delivery not meeting policy/procedure requirements is identified and corrective action taken to prevent recurrence.	❏ ❏ ❏ ❏ ❏ 20 40 60 80 100	
TX21. There is no indication from review of medical records or customer complaints that known nonconforming service occurred nor were any nonconforming medical products or supplies released or found in use.		❏ ❏ ❏ ❏ ❏ 20 40 60 80 100
TX22. Procedures exist that cover the formal review and disposition of nonconforming service and/or medical products or supplies.	❏ ❏ ❏ ❏ ❏ 20 40 60 80 100	
TX23. Records of all nonconforming service or medical products and supplies are kept and are available.	❏ ❏ ❏ ❏ ❏ 20 40 60 80 100	

Quality System Infrastructure

8 Measurement, analysis and improvement 8.3 Control of nonconforming product (Control of Nonconforming Service)	Documentation	Implementation
TX24. Observations and discussions with employees indicate that procedures and/or protocols for a formal review and disposition of nonconforming service, medical equipment, products, or supplies is consistently followed and that corrective actions taken continue to meet the needs of patients/customers and the overall organization.		☐ ☐ ☐ ☐ ☐ 20 40 60 80 100
7 Product realization **7.6 Control of monitoring and measuring devices**		
TX25. Procedures exist that document how assessment, examination, measurement, and test equipment is identified, maintained, and calibrated to ensure that measurement uncertainty is known.	☐ ☐ ☐ ☐ ☐ 20 40 60 80 100	
TX26. Procedures indicate the appropriate actions to take whenever equipment is found to be out of calibration.	☐ ☐ ☐ ☐ ☐ 20 40 60 80 100	
TX27. Records are available and maintained by biomedical or the lab that indicate the dates and results of all calibrations within specified periods of time. Records indicate the actions taken when equipment was found to be out of acceptable ranges.	☐ ☐ ☐ ☐ ☐ 20 40 60 80 100	
TX28. Centralized calibration records and labels on equipment indicate that calibration intervals are consistently on schedule and few instances of equipment out of calibration are noted.		☐ ☐ ☐ ☐ ☐ 20 40 60 80 100
TX29. Every instance of equipment out of calibration had a careful investigation of potential negative clinical effects. Effective remedial action was observed to prevent recurrence.		☐ ☐ ☐ ☐ ☐ 20 40 60 80 100
6 Resource management **6.2.2 Competence, awareness and training**		
TX30. Procedures are established to identify all training needs of personnel whose jobs affect service quality.	☐ ☐ ☐ ☐ ☐ 20 40 60 80 100	
TX31. Records of training needs and training received are readily available.	☐ ☐ ☐ ☐ ☐ 20 40 60 80 100	
TX32. Training records indicate that analysis of training needs is kept up to date and training, licensure, credentials, and qualifications are current.		☐ ☐ ☐ ☐ ☐ 20 40 60 80 100

Quality System Infrastructure

Section Scoring Sheet 2	Documentation	Implementation

4.2.3 Control of documents

D Score + *I* Score = ☐
Total Section
Score

Divide the section ___ = ☐
score by 10
Section
Average
Score

	Documentation	Implementation
TX1 _____	TX3 _____
TX2 _____	TX4 _____
TX5 _____	TX6 _____
TX9 _____	TX7 _____
	TX8 _____
	TX10 _____
D Score _____	*I* Score _____

7.5.4 Customer property

D Score + *I* Score = ☐
Total Section
Score

Divide the section ___ = ☐
score by 2
Section
Average
Score

TX11 _____	TX12 _____
D Score _____	*I* Score _____

7.5.3 Identification and traceability
(Patient Identification/Medical Product Traceability)

D Score + *I* Score = ☐
Total Section
Score

Divide the section ___ = ☐
score by 4
Section
Average
Score

TX13 _____	TX15 _____
TX14 _____	TX16 _____
D Score _____	*I* Score _____

7.5.3 Identification and traceability
(Assessment and Test Status)

D Score + *I* Score = ☐
Total Section
Score

Divide the section ___ = ☐
score by 2
Section
Average
Score

TX17 _____	TX18 _____
D Score _____	*I* Score _____

Quality System Infrastructure

Section Scoring Sheet 2	Documentation	Implementation
8.3 Control of nonconforming product (Control of Nonconforming Service) *D* Score + *I* Score = [　　　] Total Section Score Divide the section score by 6 = [　　　] Section Average Score	TX19 _____ TX20 _____ TX22 _____ TX23 _____ *D* Score _____	TX21 _____ TX24 _____ *I* Score _____
7.6 Control of monitoring and measuring devices *D* Score + *I* Score = [　　　] Total Section Score Divide the section score by 5 = [　　　] Section Average Score	TX25 _____ TX26 _____ TX27 _____ *D* Score _____	TX28 _____ TX29 _____ *I* Score _____
6.2.2 Competence, awareness and training *D* Score + *I* Score = [　　　] Total Section Score Divide the section score by 3 = [　　　] Section Average Score	TX30 _____ TX31 _____ *D* Score _____	TX32 _____ *I* Score _____

Process Management in Quality Organizations

7.2 Customer-related processes (Contracts, Orders and/or Consents)	Documentation	Implementation
PM1. Written procedures exist for reviewing all orders, consents, contracts, or customer questions to assure adequate definition of customer/patient requirements. The ability to satisfy these requirements, and methods to resolve differences and difficulties also exist.	☐ ☐ ☐ ☐ ☐ 20 40 60 80 100	
PM2. Procedures for reviewing customer orders are followed consistently, and records are maintained to demonstrate compliance, including names of reviewers if specified.		☐ ☐ ☐ ☐ ☐ 20 40 60 80 100
7 Product realization **7.3 Design and development** **7.3.1 Design and development planning**		
PM3. Procedures covering the generation of plans of care, nursing plans, minimum data sets, and clinical pathways exist.	☐ ☐ ☐ ☐ ☐ 20 40 60 80 100	
PM4. Plans for designing and developing plans of care, nursing plans, clinical pathways, minimum data sets, and other activities are generated and followed or updated as necessary.		☐ ☐ ☐ ☐ ☐ 20 40 60 80 100
PM5. Organizational and technical interfaces between different functions within the organization that have input into the design plans are defined.	☐ ☐ ☐ ☐ ☐ 20 40 60 80 100	
PM6. Information regarding the design is documented, transmitted, and regularly reviewed.		☐ ☐ ☐ ☐ ☐ 20 40 60 80 100
7.3.2 Design and development inputs		
PM7. Procedures are available describing and guiding staff as to what, where, when, and how care is to be provided to the patient during the delivery of care. Clinical care input requirements are identified, documented, and reviewed for adequacy.	☐ ☐ ☐ ☐ ☐ 20 40 60 80 100	
PM8. Care plan input requirement documents are on file and easily accessible.	☐ ☐ ☐ ☐ ☐ 20 40 60 80 100	
PM9. Documents and records indicate that procedures for reviewing input requirements are consistently followed.		☐ ☐ ☐ ☐ ☐ 20 40 60 80 100
7.3.3 Design and development outputs		
PM10. Procedures describe how the clinical input requirements are transformed into clinical care outputs. The ensuing results are the plan of care, nursing plans, completed minimum data sets, clinical pathways, and interventions.	☐ ☐ ☐ ☐ ☐ 20 40 60 80 100	
PM11. Documentation of design outputs (plan of care, nursing plans, clinical pathways, interventions, minimum data sets, etc.) is maintained and easily accessible.	☐ ☐ ☐ ☐ ☐ 20 40 60 80 100	

Process Management in Quality Organizations

7.3.3 Design and development outputs	Documentation	Implementation
PM12. A review of design outputs, change notices, customer complaints, and internal audit reports indicates consistent adherence to organizational standards for design output (plan of care, nursing plans, clinical pathways, interventions, minimum data sets, etc.)		☐ ☐ ☐ ☐ ☐ 20 40 60 80 100
7.3.4 Design and development review		
PM13. At appropriate stages of designing plans of care, nursing plans, clinical pathways, minimum data sets, interventions, or other design activities, formal documented reviews and assessments are conducted.	☐ ☐ ☐ ☐ ☐ 20 40 60 80 100	
PM14. Records of design reviews are maintained that demonstrate effective service delivery and the expected clinical outcomes.		☐ ☐ ☐ ☐ ☐ 20 40 60 80 100
7.3.5 Design and development verification		
PM15. Planning, staffing, and conducting design verification is described in formalized procedures.	☐ ☐ ☐ ☐ ☐ 20 40 60 80 100	
PM16. Results of design plan verification activities, ensuring that the proposed plan inputs (diagnosis) are meeting the outputs (interventions taken), are kept on file and readily accessible.		☐ ☐ ☐ ☐ ☐ 20 40 60 80 100
PM17. Results of design verification activities and design verification records confirm that verification procedures are followed consistently.		☐ ☐ ☐ ☐ ☐ 20 40 60 80 100
7.3.6 Design and development validation		
PM18. Procedures exist that define methods ensuring that plans of care, clinical pathways, minimum data sets, and other design activities are verified as meeting the patient's defined needs.	☐ ☐ ☐ ☐ ☐ 20 40 60 80 100	
PM19. Care plans are validated as meeting the patient's needs prior to the patient's discharge— (design input) diagnosis + (design output) interventions = (design validation) desired output.		☐ ☐ ☐ ☐ ☐ 20 40 60 80 100
7.3.7 Control of design and development changes		
PM20. Written procedures are available covering changes to nursing plans and plans of care including identification, documentation, review, and approval.	☐ ☐ ☐ ☐ ☐ 20 40 60 80 100	
PM21. Procedures for handling such changes are followed consistently, and there are few instances of problems caused by lack of control over nursing plan or plan of care changes.	☐ ☐ ☐ ☐ ☐ 20 40 60 80 100	
7.4 Purchasing		
PM22. Procedures exist that describe how subcontractors or suppliers are selected. Records are maintained that identify acceptable subcontractors or suppliers.	☐ ☐ ☐ ☐ ☐ 20 40 60 80 100	

Process Management in Quality Organizations

7.4 Purchasing	Documentation	Implementation
PM23. Purchase orders are consistently issued to subcontractors or suppliers whose names appear on the list of acceptable parties.		☐ ☐ ☐ ☐ ☐ 20 40 60 80 100
7.4.1 Purchasing process		
PM24. Procedures are available to assure that purchasing documents adequately describe products or services being ordered. Procedures describe how these documents are reviewed and approved prior to release.	☐ ☐ ☐ ☐ ☐ 20 40 60 80 100	
PM25. There are few changes to purchase orders that were caused by incomplete and inaccurate information on the original order.		☐ ☐ ☐ ☐ ☐ 20 40 60 80 100
7.1 Planning of product realization		
PM26. Documented procedures describe how to identify, plan, document, implement, and control all processes that directly affect service delivery.	☐ ☐ ☐ ☐ ☐ 20 40 60 80 100	
PM27. Current process descriptions and guidance documents are readily available to all who need them.		☐ ☐ ☐ ☐ ☐ 20 40 60 80 100
PM28. Controlled conditions exist for ensuring that processes follow prescribed regulatory requirements within defined environmental conditions and that equipment maintenance is carried out. Processes such as infection control (BBPs) are effective and followed.		☐ ☐ ☐ ☐ ☐ 20 40 60 80 100
7.4.3 Verification of purchased product (Receiving Inspection of Medical Supplies/Equipment and Assessment and Examination of Patients/Lab/Pathology)		
PM29. Procedures describe the protocols surrounding PAT, admissions of patients, receiving inspections, and verifications of purchased medical supplies upon receipt.	☐ ☐ ☐ ☐ ☐ 20 40 60 80 100	
PM30. Records are available of preadmission testing, admission of patients, and examination of preadmission test results upon, or prior to, admissions.		☐ ☐ ☐ ☐ ☐ 20 40 60 80 100
PM31. The preadmission assessments or tests and the records to be established are detailed in the policies, procedures, protocols, or instructions.	☐ ☐ ☐ ☐ ☐ 20 40 60 80 100	
PM32. Procedures detail the requirements for verification and inspection of medical supplies during receiving/incoming inspection.	☐ ☐ ☐ ☐ ☐ 20 40 60 80 100	
PM33. Procedures and nursing plans of care describe what assessments and examinations must be conducted.	☐ ☐ ☐ ☐ ☐ 20 40 60 80 100	
PM34. Records indicate what assessments, examinations, and/or tests have been carried out.		☐ ☐ ☐ ☐ ☐ 20 40 60 80 100

Process Management in Quality Organizations

7.4.3 Verification of purchased product (Receiving Inspection of Medical Supplies/Equipment and Assessment and Examination of Patients/Lab/Pathology)	Documentation	Implementation
PM35. Physician orders indicate which examinations, tests, or lab work are to be conducted for patients.		☐ ☐ ☐ ☐ ☐ 20 40 60 80 100
PM36. Records indicate what physician-ordered tests, lab work, and examinations have been carried out and when.		☐ ☐ ☐ ☐ ☐ 20 40 60 80 100
8.2.4 Monitoring and measurement of product (Assessment and Examination of Patients/Lab/Pathology)		
PM37. Procedures covering assessment, examination, and testing are described either in policy manuals or in separate documentation.	☐ ☐ ☐ ☐ ☐ 20 40 60 80 100	
PM38. Inpatient and outpatient records of assessments, examinations, and tests are readily available.		☐ ☐ ☐ ☐ ☐ 20 40 60 80 100
PM39. A combination of clinical process controls and physician-ordered testing effectively catches most clinical problems close to the source, and few problems occur or are detected at, or after, final discharge.		☐ ☐ ☐ ☐ ☐ 20 40 60 80 100
PM40. Procedures for final patient assessment or examination, education, and testing prior to discharge are maintained and are available.	☐ ☐ ☐ ☐ ☐ 20 40 60 80 100	
PM41. Final assessment, examination, and test records are readily available.		☐ ☐ ☐ ☐ ☐ 20 40 60 80 100
PM42. Results of the final discharge assessment or examinations and patient education are documented and assure that the patients understand what they are required to do to prevent readmission.		☐ ☐ ☐ ☐ ☐ 20 40 60 80 100
7.5.5 Preservation of product		
PM43. Procedures to prevent damage or deterioration of materials or supplies during handling, storage, packaging, and delivery are available. (pharmacy, lab, blood bank, patient handling, etc.)	☐ ☐ ☐ ☐ ☐ 20 40 60 80 100	
PM44. Records are maintained to demonstrate that the procedures are effective.		☐ ☐ ☐ ☐ ☐ 20 40 60 80 100
7.5 Production and service provision		
PM45. Where applicable, procedures exist to ensure that customer/patient follow-up visits are completed as scheduled by the physician.	☐ ☐ ☐ ☐ ☐ 20 40 60 80 100	
PM46. Records of follow-up visits are maintained. Schedules are made and service provided with positive patient outcomes in mind.		☐ ☐ ☐ ☐ ☐ 20 40 60 80 100
PM47. Follow-up visit procedures are effective at preventing service quality problems and creating positive patient outcomes.	☐ ☐ ☐ ☐ ☐ 20 40 60 80 100	

Process Management in Quality Organizations

Section Scoring Sheet 3	Documentation	Implementation
7.2 Customer related processes (Review of Contracts, Orders, and Consents) *D* Score + *I* Score = [＿＿＿＿] 　　　　Total Section 　　　　　Score Divide the section = [＿＿＿＿] 　score by 2 　　　　Section 　　　　Average 　　　　Score	PM1　＿＿＿＿ *D* Score ＿＿＿	PM2　＿＿＿＿ *I* Score ＿＿＿
7.3 Design and development *D* Score + *I* Score = [＿＿＿＿] 　　　　Total Section 　　　　　Score Divide the section = [＿＿＿＿] 　score by 19 　　　　Section 　　　　Average 　　　　Score	PM3　＿＿＿＿ PM5　＿＿＿＿ PM7　＿＿＿＿ PM8　＿＿＿＿ PM10　＿＿＿ PM11　＿＿＿ PM13　＿＿＿ PM15　＿＿＿ PM18　＿＿＿ PM20　＿＿＿ PM21　＿＿＿ *D* Score ＿＿＿	PM4　＿＿＿＿ PM6　＿＿＿＿ PM9　＿＿＿＿ PM12　＿＿＿ PM14　＿＿＿ PM16　＿＿＿ PM17　＿＿＿ PM19　＿＿＿ *I* Score ＿＿＿
7.4 Purchasing and 7.4.1 Purchasing process *D* Score + *I* Score = [＿＿＿＿] 　　　　Total Section 　　　　　Score Divide the section = [＿＿＿＿] 　score by 4 　　　　Section 　　　　Average 　　　　Score	PM22　＿＿＿ PM24　＿＿＿ *D* Score ＿＿＿	PM23　＿＿＿ PM25　＿＿＿ *I* Score ＿＿＿
7.1 Planning of product realization *D* Score + *I* Score = [＿＿＿＿] 　　　　Total Section 　　　　　Score Divide the section = [＿＿＿＿] 　score by 3 　　　　Section 　　　　Average 　　　　Score	PM26　＿＿＿ *D* Score ＿＿＿	PM27　＿＿＿ PM28　＿＿＿ *I* Score ＿＿＿

Process Management in Quality Organizations

Section Scoring Sheet 3	Documentation	Implementation
7.4.3 Verification of purchased product (Receiving Inspection of Medical Supplies and Assessment of Patients/Lab/Pathology) *D* Score + *I* Score = ☐ Total Section Score Divide the section score by 14 = ☐ Section Average Score	PM29 ____ PM31 ____ PM32 ____ PM33 ____ PM37 ____ PM40 ____ *D* Score ____	PM30 ____ PM34 ____ PM35 ____ PM36 ____ PM38 ____ PM39 ____ PM41 ____ PM42 ____ *I* Score ____
7.5.5 Preservation of product *D* Score + *I* Score = ☐ Total Section Score Divide the section score by 2 = ☐ Section Average Score	PM43 ____ *D* Score ____	PM44 ____ *I* Score ____
7.5 Production and service provision *D* Score + *I* Score = ☐ Total Section Score Divide the section score by 3 = ☐ Section Average Score	PM45 ____ PM46 ____ *D* Score ____	PM47 ____ *I* Score ____

Final Scoring Sheet

	Documentation	Implementation
Score Sheet 1 **Leadership and Quality Improvement**	Section Average Score	
5 Management responsibility	_____	
4.2.1 General and 4.2.2 Quality manual	_____	
8.2.2 Internal audit	_____	
4.2.3 Control of documents	_____	
8.5.2 Corrective action and 8.5.3 Preventive action	_____	
8.4 Analysis of data	_____	
Score Sheet 2 **Quality System Infrastructure**		
4.2.3 Control of documents	_____	
7.5.4 Customer property	_____	
7.5.3 Identification and traceability	_____	
7.5.3 Assessment exams and test status	_____	
8.3 Control of nonconforming product	_____	
7.6 Control of monitoring and measuring devices	_____	
6.2.2 Competence, awareness and training	_____	
Score Sheet 3 **Process Management in Quality Organizations**		
7.2 Customer related processes	_____	
7.3 Design and development	_____	
7.4 Purchasing and 7.4.1 Purchasing process	_____	
7.1 Planning of product realization	_____	
7.4.3 Verification of purchased product	_____	
7.5.5 Preservation of product	_____	
7.5 Production and service provision	_____	
Add columns and enter here	☞	
Divide total score by 20 This score represents your percentage of readiness for ISO 9001 certification.	☞	%

Appendix B

Sample Quality Systems Manual and Procedures

This appendix contains a sample manual and the six procedures required by ISO 9001:2000. The samples allow a healthcare organization to begin the implementation process toward ISO 9001:2000 registration. However, the manual and procedures alone will not be enough for the healthcare organization to meet all of the requirements of the ISO 9001:2000 standard, nor will certification be granted by simply editing these documents and using them. The sample manual and procedures only provide a starting point for the organization.

It is highly recommended that assistance from qualified consultants be sought prior to actual implementation of the quality management system; other procedures, in addition to those in the appendix, are needed to be successful. When seeking guidance from consultants, a healthcare organization should consider two important factors: the consulting firm should be ISO 9001:2000 certified, and the firm should have experience in assisting other healthcare organizations in achieving ISO 9001:2000 certification. There are thousands of consulting firms to choose from, but only a small handful meet both these criteria. If additional guidance or assistance is required, please feel free to contact Bryce Carson at authors@asq.org.

Quality Paradigms Medical Center	Quality Systems Manual Page 1 of 27
ISO 9001:2000 Quality Systems Manual	Issued: Revised: Supersedes:

Quality Systems Manual
for
Quality Paradigms Medical Center

1 Process Management Way
Continual Improvement, New Jersey 07823

Quality Paradigms Medical Center ISO 9001:2000 Quality Systems Manual	Quality Systems Manual Page 2 of 27
	Issued: Revised: Supersedes:

Document Authorization

Dr. Frank Jones, President   Date

Jackie Franks, VP, Operations   Date

Joanna Jakes, VP, Marketing & Development   Date

Change Record

Rev. Date	Responsible Person	Description of Change

Quality Paradigms Medical Center **ISO 9001:2000 Quality Systems Manual**	Quality Systems Manual Page 3 of 27
	Issued: Revised: Supersedes:

Quality Systems Manual
Table of contents

1 Definitions 5
2 Scope 6
3 Introduction 7
4 Quality management system 7
   4.1 General requirements 8
   4.2 Documentation requirements 8
      4.2.1 General 8
      4.2.2 Quality manual 8
      4.2.3 Control of documents 8
      4.2.4 Control of records 9
5 Management responsibility 9
   5.1 Management commitment 9
   5.2 Customer focus 10
   5.3 Quality policy 10
   5.4 Planning 10
      5.4.1 Quality objectives 10
      5.4.2 Quality management system planning 11
   5.5 Responsibility, authority and communication 12
      5.5.1 Responsibility and authority 12
      5.5.2 Management representative 13
      5.5.3 Internal communication 14
   5.6 Management review 14
6 Resource management 14
   6.1 Provision of resources 14
   6.2 Human resources 15
      6.2.1 General 15
      6.2.2 Competence, awareness, and training 15
   6.3 Infrastructure 15
   6.4 Work environment 15
7 Product realization 15
   7.1 Planning of product realization 15
   7.2 Customer-related processes 16
      7.2.1 Determination of requirements related to the product 16
      7.2.2 Review of patient/customer requirements 16
      7.2.3 Customer communication 17
   7.3 Design and development 17
      7.3.1 Design and development planning 17
      7.3.2 Design and development inputs 17

Quality Paradigms Medical Center	Quality Systems Manual Page 4 of 27
ISO 9001:2000 Quality Systems Manual	Issued: Revised: Supersedes:

7.3.3 Design and development outputs 18
7.3.4 Design and development review 18
7.3.5 Design and development verification 18
7.3.6 Design and development validation 18
7.3.7 Control of design and development changes 18
7.4 Purchasing 19
   7.4.1 Purchasing process 19
   7.4.2 Purchasing information 19
   7.4.3 Verification of purchased product 19
7.5 Service delivery 19
   7.5.1 Control of service delivery 19
   7.5.2 Validation of processes for production and service provision 20
   7.5.3 Identification and traceability 20
   7.5.4 Customer property 21
   7.5.5 Handling, packaging, storage, and protection—Caring for patients,
       medical products and supplies 21
7.6 Control of monitoring and measuring devices 22
8 Measurement, analysis and improvement 24
8.1 General 24
8.2 Monitoring and measurement 24
   8.2.1 Patient/customer satisfaction 24
   8.2.2 Internal audit 24
   8.2.3 Monitoring and measurement of processes 25
   8.2.4 Monitoring and measurement of product 25
8.3 Control of nonconforming product 25
8.4 Analysis of data 25
8.5 Improvement 26
   8.5.1 Continual improvement 26
   8.5.2 Corrective action 26
   8.5.3 Preventive action 27

Quality Paradigms Medical Center	Quality Systems Manual Page 5 of 27
ISO 9001:2000 Quality Systems Manual	Issued: Revised: Supersedes:

1 Definitions

Top Management: President and board of directors have authorized the vice president of operations to function as top management for the quality management system.

ISO Team: Department managers, various departmental employees, Management representative, director of performance improvement, and vice president of operations.

Management Representative: Person designated to ensure that the quality system is established, implemented, and maintained in accordance with the ISO 9001:2000 standard, and who reports on quality system performance for management review as a basis for improving the quality system.

Departments within the Quality Paradigms Medical Center:

Administration	Nutritional Services
Risk Management/Corporate Compliance	Plant Operations
Nursing Administration	Environmental Services
Community Education	Linen Services
Occupational Health	Registration
Medical/Surgical	Billing
Obstetrics	Accounting
Critical Care Unit	Information Services
Respiratory Therapy	Social Services
Cardiopulmonary Rehabilitation	Volunteer Services
Surgery	Health Information Management
Emergency Department	Case Management
Central Services	Medical Staff Services
Laboratory	Materials Management
Cardiopulmonary Diagnostics	Telecommunications
Radiology	Planning/Marketing/Fund Development
Pharmacy	Human Resources
Anesthesiology	Medical Control Authority
Fitness & Rehab	Emergency Medical Services

Controlled document: Document currently approved for use in the quality system.

Obsolete document: Document that has been discontinued or superseded by revision.

Record: Information to be input in a controlled document.

Nonconformance: Failure to comply with the applicable standard or procedure.

Customer: Internal customers, patients, physicians, guests, community, and other interested stakeholders.

Quality Paradigms Medical Center ISO 9001:2000 Quality Systems Manual	Quality Systems Manual Page 6 of 27
	Issued: Revised: Supersedes:

Process: Flow of work defined in policies, procedures, protocols, instructions, or a simple list of steps. System procedures at Quality Paradigms Medical Center (QPMC) are defined as *Policies* and *Procedures.*

Stakeholder: Anyone who has a vested interest in the welfare of QPMC.

Policy: Overall statement of what is to be accomplished.

Procedure: Guideline to implementing the policy statement.

Protocol: What action steps are required to accomplish a specified task.

Competency: Skills required to complete a job.

Job Description: Lists the following characteristics for each position

Desired performance of an individual
Required qualifications
Expected behaviors
Scope of responsibility
Physical requirements
Potential environmental factors

Benchmark: Assessment of where QPMC is compared to institutions of similar size and capabilities.

Quality Record: Documentation that demonstrates conformance to the requirements of a quality system.

2 Scope

This manual describes the quality system requirements for services provided by Quality Paradigms Medical Center. Services include:

- Inpatient and outpatient surgery
- Diagnostic laboratory
- Medical imaging and nuclear medicine
- Mammography
- Critical care unit
- Obstetrics
- Pediatrics
- General medical/surgical patient education
- Social services
- Physical therapy
- Speech therapy
- Diagnostic respiratory therapy
- Emergency department
- Cardiac rehabilitation
- Wellness center
- Ambulance service
- Dietary counseling
- Cardiopulmonary
- Occupational therapy
- Pharmacy services
- Chemotherapy

Quality Paradigms Medical Center **ISO 9001:2000 Quality Systems Manual**	Quality Systems Manual Page 7 of 27
	Issued: Revised: Supersedes:

Service requirements are specified between QPMC and its physicians, patients, vendors, and customers through multiple arrangements: service contracts, fee for service agreements, grants, credentials, and privileging.

Hospital services and compliance with contractual and regulatory standards are controlled to ensure the delivery of quality service to satisfy all specified requirements.

This manual provides a description of the quality management system in accordance with the ISO 9001:2000 requirements and serves as a reference for implementation and maintenance of QPMC's quality management system.

3 Introduction

QPMC, with more than 3000 employees, is located in northwestern New Jersey. QPMC is headquartered at 1 Process Management Way, Continual Improvement, New Jersey 07823. QPMC provides a full continuum of healthcare services. The Medical Center is licensed for 500 beds and serves approximately 458,000 people in Warren and Sussex counties. QPMC is accredited by the State of New Jersey Department of Health.

This quality systems manual is controlled in accordance with Clause 4.2.3 of the ISO 9001:2000 standard that refers to control of documents.

4 Quality management system

4.1 General requirements

Quality Paradigms Medical Center ensures that services delivered comply with customer requirements and expectations by defining and managing the healthcare service delivery processes. QPMC's quality management system addresses all requirements and elements of the ISO 9001:2000 standard. All processes necessary for delivery of quality services and compliance with patient/customer requirements are defined, implemented, maintained, controlled, and continually improved. Criteria and methods necessary for effective operation and process control are determined and implemented; processes are monitored and analyzed as necessary.

Services and/or supporting activities that are outsourced are controlled. Such controls are defined in the quality system.

Processes are described in order to:

- Facilitate understanding of the work flow

- Facilitate the understanding of responsibility lines

- Demonstrate the complexity and importance of the interactions involved in work performance

- Demonstrate how the design of the work flow relates to the achievement of quality outcomes including continually improving the quality management system

Quality Paradigms Medical Center ISO 9001:2000 Quality Systems Manual	Quality Systems Manual Page 8 of 27
	Issued: Revised: Supersedes:

- Demonstrate compliance with applicable standards and legal/regulatory requirements

- Demonstrate how the organization controls its processes at every level of the management structure

4.2 Documentation requirements

4.2.1 General

Quality management system documents at QPMC are defined at four different levels within the organization's quality management structure. The four levels are outlined as follows:

Quality Systems Manual (Tier 1) describes the elements and scope of QPMC's quality management system.

Quality System Procedures (Tier 2) describe the implementation of the requirements of the quality management system for the entire organization. These are hard copy controlled documents.

Policies and Procedures (Tier 3) describe specific practice and controls for necessary activities. These are electronic documents located by department.

Procedures are drafted where the absence of such procedures would adversely affect healthcare service quality and delivery.

Instructions, Protocols, and Forms (Tier 4) describe details of practice and control specific activities.

4.2.2 Quality manual

This quality systems manual demonstrates QPMC's application and scope of the ISO 9001:2000 standard and all of its elements. Supporting system-level procedures (Tier 2) are referenced on the master list of system procedures published with the quality systems manual. The manual describes the interaction between the processes of the quality management system.

4.2.3 Control of documents

All data and documents relating to the quality system, including this manual, are controlled as described by documented procedure. The quality policy and quality objectives are documented and controlled. Documents of external origin are identified, and their distribution is controlled to ensure that the most current documents are used.

All quality system documents are reviewed and approved prior to issue. They are reviewed, updated, and reapproved as necessary.

Quality Paradigms Medical Center **ISO 9001:2000 Quality Systems Manual**	Quality Systems Manual Page 9 of 27
	Issued: Revised: Supersedes:

All documents are controlled to ensure that only current versions of documents are available where activities are performed. One signed and/or initialed hard copy of documents is maintained by administration. This copy contains the official signed and/or initialed up-to-date version for state regulatory purposes.

Obsolete documents are removed from all points of use. When retained, these documents are clearly identified and placed in a specified file cabinet to prevent unintended use.

Master lists of documents are maintained in an electronic policy and procedure cabinet and protocol cabinets for each department (database). Within the cabinet, there are drawers for each department's policies and procedures.

Master lists comprise a series of indexes containing document name and issue date. Quality system documents are legible, readily identifiable, and retrievable.

4.2.4 Control of records

Records are identified for processes in the quality management system. The records demonstrate conformance to the requirements and show that the quality system is working effectively. A quality system procedure defines the identification, storage, retrieval, protection, retention time, and disposition of records.

5 Management responsibility

5.1 Management commitment

The vice president of operations has been authorized by the president and board of directors to function as top management for the quality management system. The vice president of operations has a reporting relationship with the president and board of directors.

The quality management system described herein is evidence of the commitment of top management. Developing and implementing a quality management system that is capable of continuous improvement is a task accomplished only in a supportive environment from executive management. Further evidence of top management's commitment is demonstrated by continued attention from the vice president of operations to the importance of meeting both customer needs and the many and varied requirements of statutes and regulations, a quality policy and quality objectives that are defined and relevant, provision of resources necessary for the needs of an effective quality management system, and the establishment of a review process for the quality system that encompasses top management and all levels of management in a defined plan.

The vice president of operations has appointed an ISO team to oversee the establishment and implementation of the quality management system.

Quality Paradigms Medical Center ISO 9001:2000 Quality Systems Manual	Quality Systems Manual Page 10 of 27
	Issued: Revised: Supersedes:

5.2 Customer focus

The ISO team appointed by the vice president of operations ensures that patient/customer needs, requirements, and expectations are properly determined and met. The ultimate goal of this effort is to enhance customer satisfaction and confidence.

5.3 Quality policy

QPMC's mission is as follows:

> Strive to improve the healthcare status of the community and to deliver healthcare to individuals in a way that provides local and regional access to quality care and advocates respect for the individual, appropriate use of resources, and cost-effective services

This mission statement has been adopted as the current quality statement or quality policy. The quality policy is communicated through newsletters, staff meetings, training opportunities, and other appropriate forums. All employees are encouraged and required to embrace this policy.

The ISO team has the responsibility to ensure that QPMC's quality policy:

- Is relevant to the nature of services provided by the organization and to the needs and expectations of its customers

- Underscores the organization's commitment to meeting applicable requirements and standards

- Underscores the organization's dedication to continual quality improvement

- Provides a framework for establishing and reviewing the organization's quality goals and objectives

- Is communicated, understood, and implemented at all levels of the organization

- Is reviewed on a regular basis for continuing suitability and relevance to the overall purpose of the organization

The quality policy is a controlled document in accordance with Section 4.2.3 of this manual.

5.4 Planning

5.4.1 Quality objectives

Quality objectives are established for relevant functions of the organization. These objectives are consistent with the intent of QPMC's quality policy, reinforce the organization's

Quality Paradigms Medical Center ISO 9001:2000 Quality Systems Manual	Quality Systems Manual Page 11 of 27
	Issued: Revised: Supersedes:

commitment to continual quality improvement, are relevant to the nature of services provided, and are measurable.

5.4.2 Quality management system planning

QPMC's quality planning is designed to support the achievement of its quality objectives and promote continuous quality improvement. QPMC's quality planning at the executive level addresses all the requirements and factors that have some bearing on the organization's mission and scope of services, which includes:

- Customer requirements and satisfaction

- Market trends or needs

- Efficiency of its service structure within the quality management system

- Labor and employment issues

- Procurement of resources

- Assignment of resources

- Growth issues

- Effectiveness of services provided

- Relationship with funding sources

- Compliance with applicable standards and requirements

- Continual improvement of the quality management system

- Relationship to affiliates

- Community needs

- Legal requirements

Quality planning at departmental levels is developed in order to support the overall quality planning of the organization.

QPMC's quality planning covers:

- Processes required for the quality management system

- Identification of processes and resources needed to achieve desired results

- Identification of quality requirements at defined stages of service delivery

- Verification activities such as quality audits

- Identification and control of necessary records

Quality Paradigms Medical Center **ISO 9001:2000 Quality Systems Manual**	Quality Systems Manual Page 12 of 27
	Issued: Revised: Supersedes:

Quality planning controls organizational and process changes thus ensuring that the quality management system is maintained at all times.

5.5 Responsibility, authority and communication

5.5.1 Responsibility and authority

Roles and responsibilities within the organization are defined by top management and clearly communicated to employees. Responsibility and authority over each organizational function as well as its interrelationship with other functions within the organization is clearly delineated to facilitate effective quality management.

The president is responsible to communicate to the board of directors for its support in the quality initiatives. The president also provides the necessary resources to support quality, nonclinical, and clinical initiatives.

The executive council is comprised of the president and vice presidents. This council oversees all operations at QPMC.

The vice president of operations has the ultimate responsibility for the overall quality system and its operational effectiveness. The vice president of operations is charged with these responsibilities:

- Maintaining the organizational structure that controls and manages all the elements of the quality system.

- Assigning the responsibility and authority to ensure that the quality system is understood, implemented, and maintained.

- Identifying and providing adequate resources for management, performance of work, and verification activities including internal quality audits. The vice president of operations ensures that adequate resources are assigned to implement the quality program and to achieve its objectives.

Department managers are responsible for:

- Ensuring that services provided conform to specified standards and customer requirements

- Ensuring that nonconformities in the service delivery system are properly identified, recorded, corrected, and prevented

- Controlling further processing and delivery of service until any identified deficiency or unsatisfactory condition has been corrected

- Verifying the effectiveness of corrective action plans

The department managers, in consultation with the vice president of operations, are responsible for identifying resources required for the provision of services in their

Quality Paradigms Medical Center	Quality Systems Manual Page 13 of 27
ISO 9001:2000 Quality Systems Manual	Issued: Revised: Supersedes:

departments (hiring and training of staff, purchasing of equipment, and so on). Assignment of the required resources is the responsibility of department managers or the vice president of operations as defined by applicable QPMC policies. The department managers are responsible for the implementation of processes that ensure compliance with any applicable requirement or standard.

The vice president of operations is responsible for operational decisions related to quality and the quality management system. The management representative reports directly to the vice president of operations. The management representative evaluates the quality system and reports the results of the evaluation to the vice president of operations who reports the findings to the PI committee for systems analysis and to the executive council and the board during management review. The management representative is assisted by the internal audit coordinator, who oversees the scheduling, implementation, and follow-up of internal audit activities, and an administrative assistant who inputs, tracks, and assists in trending the audit findings.

The ISO team, headed by the management representative, establishes and implements the quality system.

QPMC employees are responsible for performing work in accordance with applicable quality standards, procedures, instructions, and protocols and complying with the quality policy.

5.5.2 Management representative

The management representative is appointed by the president and/or the vice president of operations.

The management representative has the authority and responsibility to ensure that the requirements of this quality systems manual and of the entire quality management system are implemented, maintained, and continuously improved.

The management representative reports to top management on the performance of the quality management system and any need for improvement. This is accomplished through the reporting structure of the vice president of operations to the performance improvement committee, the executive council, and the board of directors.

Additionally, the management representative is responsible for promoting awareness of customer requirements throughout all levels of the organization. This awareness shall include:

- Patient requirements defined through the physician order process for each patient

- Performance improvement plans

- Nursing plans of care (care plans)

- Community surveys and results distribution

Quality Paradigms Medical Center **ISO 9001:2000 Quality Systems Manual**	Quality Systems Manual Page 14 of 27
	Issued: Revised: Supersedes:

- Training sessions with medical center employees

- Instructions, protocols, and memoranda

5.5.3 Internal communication

Communication throughout the organization concerning quality issues is the responsibility of the vice president of operations. Communication is achieved by several methods. E-mails are a tool used by all employees for communicating every issue including quality. In addition, bimonthly manager meetings are held to address any pertinent issue and to hold a forum where concerns are addressed by employees to top management and from top management to employees. Managers hold departmental meetings to communicate to their employees as needed. Managers also meet with the appropriate vice president or director on a monthly basis.

5.6 Management review

The vice president of operations, in the role of management representative, reports to the entire executive council regarding the effectiveness of the quality management system as part of the annual review of the organization's quality management system. This review is held to establish or review the quality policy, quality objectives, and quality planning, maintain and continuously improve the quality management system, and ensure that proper resources are available. Records are maintained for management review.

Inputs to the management review process include reports from the departmental managers on service performance analysis, results of internal and external audits, status and results of corrective and preventive actions, customer feedback, follow-up actions from previous management reviews, and any other relevant information that determines the effectiveness of the quality system and its continuing suitability. This activity also includes a review of the quality policy to ensure continued relevance, identification of changing circumstances that can affect the quality system, and any recommendations for improvement that have been documented.

Outputs from the management review include actions designed to improve the effectiveness of the quality management system, actions related to improving quality of care and/or defined requirements, and actions relating to resource needs.

6 Resource management

6.1 Provision of Resources

Resources are provided in order to establish and maintain QPMC's quality management system and to satisfy customers. Resources are properly identified and assigned based on need, priority, urgency and other criteria relevant to the operation and continuous improvement of the organization's quality system.

Quality Paradigms Medical Center **ISO 9001:2000 Quality Systems Manual**	Quality Systems Manual Page 15 of 27
	Issued: Revised: Supersedes:

6.2 Human resources

6.2.1 General

Human Resources is responsible for verifying competency of employees with defined responsibilities in the quality management system based on education, training, skills, and experience. Only employees who are deemed competent are assigned responsibilities in the quality management system.

6.2.2 Competence, awareness, and training

Based on organizational responsibilities, QPMC will:

- Determine training needs and requirements for competency.

- Provide training when a need is identified.

- Evaluate effectiveness of training at prescribed intervals.

- Ensure that employees are aware of their role in the achievement of the Medical Center's quality goals and objectives.

- Maintain records for education, training, skills, and experience.

6.3 Infrastructure

Infrastructure for the QPMC organization includes work spaces and facilities, equipment including hardware and software, and supporting services needed to achieve compliance with requirements and standards for service delivery.

6.4 Work environment

Human and physical factors in the work environment are defined and implemented to ensure conformity for the healthcare service delivery.

7 Product realization

7.1 Planning of product realization

QPMC identifies plans and implements processes necessary to realize requirements for service delivery. Quality system procedures describe the sequence and interaction of activities and establish system methods and controls. Policies and procedures provide specific direction for an activity described in Tier 2 system procedures. Policies and procedures are found in the appropriate departmental drawer in the Meditech system. Outputs from quality planning are considered in identifying needed processes.

In planning process realization, QPMC:

- Defines quality objectives and service requirements

Quality Paradigms Medical Center	Quality Systems Manual Page 16 of 27
ISO 9001:2000 Quality Systems Manual	Issued: Revised: Supersedes:

- Establishes methods and practices designed to achieve consistent operation

- Determines and implements control of the process and defines methods and criteria to achieve defined service outcomes

- Verifies that the process can achieve the defined service outcomes

- Determines and implements measurement, monitoring, and follow-up activities so the process continues to achieve planned outcomes

- Ensures availability of information and data necessary for effective operation and monitoring of processes

- Maintains records of monitoring and verification activities, including appropriate measurements, to provide evidence of effective operation of processes

7.2 Customer-related processes

7.2.1 Determination of requirements related to the product

QPMC delivers healthcare services. Requirements for product are determined to be characteristics or requirements for service delivery.

Patient/customer requirements are established through the use of physician orders, patient consent forms, and/or contracts for service. These requirements include both service delivery and postservice activities as applicable. There are often multiple customers for any particular service, and all requirements must be met for patients, regulatory agencies, and other stakeholders. Additional requirements may be determined and required by QPMC.

7.2.2 Review of patient/customer requirements

Patient/customer requirements are reviewed before commitment to provide services. These commitments are defined as review of physician orders, insurance requirements, preadmission testing, preanesthesia screenings, discussions regarding the services performed and the expected outcomes from those services, and so on.

Commitments are reviewed to ensure that:

- Requirements are clearly defined.

- All requirements are confirmed by the patient/customer before their acceptance.

- Differences between the service requirements of the patient/customer and the care provider are reconciled and resolved prior to performing the service.

- The organization has the ability to meet requirements for service as requested.

Both the results of the review of agreements and any follow-up actions are recorded. Where service requirements are changed, either by the patient/customer or the service

Quality Paradigms Medical Center ISO 9001:2000 Quality Systems Manual	Quality Systems Manual Page 17 of 27
	Issued: Revised: Supersedes:

provider, documentation may be amended, and all relevant personnel are made aware of the changed requirements.

7.2.3 Customer communication

In order to meet customer requirements, QPMC has established arrangements for communication with patients/customers. Communication arrangements address the following aspects:

- Information about services provided and impact of services

- Information related to modification of any service to be provided

- Patient/customer feedback about acceptability of service

7.3 Design and development

7.3.1 Design and development planning

Documented procedures are maintained to plan and control the development of care plans. Design and development planning procedures include:

- Stages of the development process

- Required reviews

- Verification and validation activities

- Responsibilities and authorities over care plan development activities

Interfaces between different groups involved in the design and development of care plans are managed so that communication is clear and effective and design responsibilities are understood. Planning outputs are updated as appropriate as the care plan design and development evolves.

7.3.2 Design and development inputs

As part of the care plan design and development process, applicable requirements are identified, defined, and properly recorded and maintained. These documented requirements include:

- Standards of identified patient/customer needs

- Applicable regulatory and legal requirements

- Requirements from previous similar care plans

- Input from employees and physician practice guidelines

- Other requirements required for development

Quality Paradigms Medical Center **ISO 9001:2000 Quality Systems Manual**	Quality Systems Manual Page 18 of 27
	Issued: Revised: Supersedes:

All requirements are reviewed for adequacy. Requirements that appear to be incomplete, ambiguous, or conflicting are resolved.

7.3.3 Design and development outputs

Outputs or outcomes of the care plan development process are recorded so that they can be compared to the input requirements. Development outcomes must meet input requirements, provide necessary information to ensure effective healthcare delivery, and define goals of the care plan that are essential to the health and safety of the patient/customer. Design output documents are approved before release.

7.3.4 Design and development review

Systematic reviews are planned and conducted at suitable stages in the design and/or development process. These reviews evaluate the content and effectiveness of the care plan in order to direct the interventions and expected patient outcomes.

Representatives from all relevant functions involved at the applicable stage of development participate in the review. Records are maintained of the review and subsequent follow-up actions.

7.3.5 Design and development verification

Design verification at QPMC is performed as part of design review. The purpose of design review and design verification is to ensure consistency between design input and output. Verification takes place when the proposed care plan is accepted by the clinical analyst. Results of verification and any follow-up are recorded and maintained.

7.3.6 Design and development validation

Care plan validation confirms that the plan is capable of meeting the specified outcome requirements. When possible, partial validation is undertaken prior to implementation of a care plan. When it is not practical to validate in advance, validation occurs at the completion of the first program outcome evaluation. The results of design validation and any follow-up activities are recorded and maintained.

7.3.7 Control of design and development changes

Modifications to the care plan are approved by authorized personnel and recorded before implementation. Where specified, stakeholders are consulted for approval.

Care plan developers determine:

- The evaluation of the effect of changes in order to promote a positive outcome

- The interaction between care plan component parts that affect patient care delivery

- The need for reverification or revalidation for the program or outcomes

Resulting review of changes and follow-up actions are recorded and maintained.

Quality Paradigms Medical Center **ISO 9001:2000 Quality Systems Manual**	Quality Systems Manual Page 19 of 27
	Issued: Revised: Supersedes:

7.4 Purchasing

7.4.1 Purchasing process

QPMC has documented and implemented procedures to ensure that all medical products, supplies, and services purchased conform to specified requirements. The type and extent of control exercised over vendors and purchased product is dependent on the effect of the product on service delivery. Vendors, suppliers, and subcontractors are evaluated and selected based on their ability to supply product in accordance with QPMC's established policies and procedures.

Vendors are selected based upon:

- Reputation of the vendor

- Ability to deliver in a timely manner

- Quality of products and services

- Competitive pricing

- Professional qualifications and/or proof of insurance for subcontracted services or certifications.

Periodic evaluation may be performed. Results of evaluations and subsequent follow-up actions are recorded and maintained.

7.4.2 Purchasing information

Purchasing documents clearly describe the product or service ordered including any associated requirements. The requirements needed for approval, qualification of product, procedures, processes, equipment, and personnel requirements are defined. Purchasing documents are reviewed and approved prior to release.

7.4.3 Verification of purchased product

Purchased items are subjected to receiving inspection to verify that the product received complies with stated requirements. If QPMC desires a vendor audit, arrangements for this requirement are specified on the purchase order.

7.5 Service delivery

7.5.1 Control of service delivery

Healthcare delivery processes are planned and controlled. This control includes:

- Information available in the workplace that describes characteristics of service delivery

Quality Paradigms Medical Center ISO 9001:2000 Quality Systems Manual	Quality Systems Manual Page 20 of 27
	Issued: Revised: Supersedes:

- Work instructions where activities are necessary for achieving conformity of service

- Use of suitable equipment

- A suitable working environment

- The availability and use of suitable measuring and monitoring equipment

- Suitable monitoring, assessment, and examination activities

- Implementing defined processes for completion of healthcare services

7.5.2 Validation of processes for production and service provision

Enhanced healthcare processes cannot be verified until after the process is fully implemented. Therefore, QPMC ensures that qualified personnel are appointed to develop and/or carry out these services. Where appropriate, these services are continuously monitored to ensure that specified standards of care are met. Surgery is defined as a process that requires continuous monitoring. Validation of processes demonstrates the organization's ability to achieve planned outcomes.

Validation activities shall include the following:

- Qualification of processes

- Qualification of equipment and personnel

- Use of appropriate procedures and protocols

- Established requirements for maintaining records of validated processes

- Revalidation of processes when critical process parameters have been changed

7.5.3 Identification and traceability

Patients are identified and tracked throughout the healthcare service delivery processes.

Traceability of implantable medical devices is a specified requirement; these and other medical products that require tracking throughout the service delivery process are identified with unique identifiers that are recorded and maintained in accordance with hospital policy and procedures.

To identify patients, medical devices, and other products requiring identification and/or traceability, QPMC utilizes these identification and traceability methods:

- The use of first and last names for patients

- Identification banding of patients

- The use of double banding of mothers and babies

- Financial identification numbers that identify each patient

Quality Paradigms Medical Center	Quality Systems Manual Page 21 of 27
ISO 9001:2000 Quality Systems Manual	Issued: Revised: Supersedes:

- The use of a social security number or equivalent identification

- The use of packing slips, purchase order numbers, incoming lot numbers, stock numbers, and catalog numbers

The use of medical record numbers is the process that identifies each patient's records.

7.5.4 Customer property

Patient/customer property may be defined as any item brought to the medical center by a patient or family. Patient property is under the control of patients while it is in their possession and is not the responsibility of QPMC. All patient/customer property that is under the control of the medical center is verified, stored, and maintained in accordance with documented procedures. Provision of appropriate areas for temporary storage of personal items does not constitute control of patient property.

Any such item that is lost, damaged, or otherwise becomes unsuitable for use is recorded and reported to the patient/customer and to the risk manager. Records are maintained.

7.5.5 Handling, packaging, storage, and protection—Caring for patients, medical products, and supplies

Medical Products and Supplies

QPMC policies and procedures ensure that all medical products and supplies are identified, handled, packaged, stored, and protected to maintain the integrity of the purchased products.

Care of Patients

Patients/customers are handled and transported in accordance with hospital policies and procedures. Employees are trained in proper techniques for the care of patients in various environments and healthcare delivery situations. This care includes issues related to the environment, safety, and patient rights.

Specific training provided for the care of patients in service processes includes:

- Patient rights and responsibilities

- CPR and first aid (as applicable)

- Universal precautions

- Fire safety, electrical, and hazardous materials

- Behavioral management plans (as applicable)

- Physical/nonphysical management (as applicable)

Quality Paradigms Medical Center	Quality Systems Manual Page 22 of 27
ISO 9001:2000 Quality Systems Manual	Issued: Revised: Supersedes:

- Specialized care needs applicable to specific patients

- Topics as determined by program needs

Employees are trained in the proper handling, maintenance, and storage of materials. Training is provided in:

- Blood-borne pathogens (BBP)

- Medication administration (as applicable).

- The right to know (MSDS)

- Confidentiality issues (HIPAA)

Storage

Designated storage areas are used to protect materials from damage or deterioration as applicable prior to use or delivery. Storage areas are secure to prevent damage or deterioration of product, pending use or delivery. Medications and hazardous materials are secured to restrict access. The condition of stored product is regularly assessed as appropriate. Proper authorization is required for removal from storage areas.

Packaging

Items are packaged to survive transportation and handling environments (sterile products and packs, storage bins, and baskets). Factors considered include fragility, environment conditions, mode of shipment, and expected length of storage. Training is provided in the proper packaging and storage of materials.

Preservation

Appropriate methods of preserving and segregating medical products and supplies are implemented and communicated. Food products are stored in appropriate storage containers to prevent spoilage.

Delivery of Materials, Equipment, and Lab Specimens

Where specified, QPMC is responsible for packaging and preserving products during transit and delivery to destination.

Transportation of Patients

Where legally or contractually specified, QPMC is responsible for the welfare of patients until transfer of responsibility.

7.6 Control of monitoring and measuring devices

Controls are established to maintain the integrity of equipment and devices used in measuring and testing.

Quality Paradigms Medical Center **ISO 9001:2000 Quality Systems Manual**	Quality Systems Manual Page 23 of 27
	Issued: Revised: Supersedes:

The plant operations manager (or other appropriate manager) schedules, calibrates, and maintains inspection, measuring, and testing devices to ensure conformity to specifications so that required measurement capability is known and is consistent with measurement requirements.

Calibration is traceable to national standards where such standards exist:

- QPMC maintains individual calibration records of all inspection, measuring, and testing devices.

- New equipment is registered and calibrated prior to use for inspection, measuring, and testing.

- Inspection, measuring, and testing equipment is identified and calibrated at prescribed intervals.

- QPMC provides employees with training in the handling, storage, and use of inspection, measuring, and testing equipment, where required, so that improper handling does not invalidate the calibration settings.

- Safeguards against inadvertent adjustments to equipment are used when applicable.

- Any product that has been tested using out-of-tolerance equipment is reinspected and corrective action is taken.

QPMC ensures that:

- Required measurements and accuracy are determined.

- Appropriate inspection, measuring, and testing instruments capable of the necessary accuracy are used.

- Inspection, measuring, and testing equipment is identified and calibrated at prescribed intervals.

- Equipment used for calibration is traceable to national standards or another standard. Where no such standards exist, the basis for the calibration will be documented.

- Calibration records contain details of the calibration process used, type of equipment, identification, location, frequency of checks, acceptance criteria, and action taken to adjust the instrument.

- Calibration stickers or calibration records identify calibration status.

- Records are maintained.

Quality Paradigms Medical Center	Quality Systems Manual Page 24 of 27
ISO 9001:2000 Quality Systems Manual	Issued: Revised: Supersedes:

- When equipment is found to be out of calibration, previous test results using the instrument are assessed to determine validity.

- Suitable environmental conditions exist for the calibration being carried out.

- Accuracy and fitness for use of the device is maintained by proper handling and storage.

- Facilities and devices are safeguarded from adjustments that would invalidate the calibration setting.

8 Measurement, analysis, and improvement

8.1 General

To ensure that QPMC's services comply with its established requirements, the medical center employs a system whereby processes and outcomes of services throughout the organization are measured, monitored, reviewed, modified, and improved as necessary. This system employs statistical techniques to gather information on specific measurement areas such as effectiveness of services provided, patient satisfaction, and stakeholder satisfaction.

8.2 Monitoring and measurement

8.2.1 Patient/customer satisfaction

QPMC has established processes for measurement, monitoring, and review of information related to the performance level of the organization. QPMC has a system to identify, quantify and qualify patient and stakeholder levels of satisfaction with the organization's services. This system includes surveys at various points of the service provision continuum, questionnaires and other inquiry formats. The system is designed to generate information that can be used for immediate modification of planned services, for modification of the structure of the organization's service components, for long-term planning, and for continual improvement of the organization's service delivery system.

8.2.2 Internal audit

QPMC has a program to audit its quality management system on a regular basis. The internal audit schedule for the various activities of the medical center is established in accordance with the significance and impact that the audited activities have on the overall quality system and in accordance with the results of previous internal audits. Each segment of the medical center and component of the quality system is audited at least annually. Auditors are independent of the area audited.

Quality Paradigms Medical Center ISO 9001:2000 Quality Systems Manual	Quality Systems Manual Page 25 of 27
	Issued: Revised: Supersedes:

QPMC maintains a system-level procedure that outlines the scope, frequency, and methodology of its internal audits. This procedure also establishes the terms of eligibility and responsibility for internal audits and the mechanism for reporting audit results to appropriate management personnel. Actions are taken in a timely manner to eliminate causes of nonconformity. Follow-up activities include verification that actions taken are effective. Records of internal audit activities are maintained.

8.2.3 Monitoring and measurement of processes

QPMC has established methods to monitor activities that demonstrate the ability of the activities to achieve planned results. Corrective action is taken when necessary.

8.2.4 Monitoring and measurement of product

Outcome measures and other indicators of service delivery are monitored to verify that requirements have been met. Records indicating the authority responsible for release of the patient or product are maintained.

8.3 Control of nonconforming product

QPMC has established methods to collect information related to the effectiveness and output of processes used in healthcare delivery. QPMC maintains a system to monitor, detect, and correct nonconformances. Every employee has the responsibility for identifying and reporting nonconformances. Notification of service nonconformities is the responsibility of area managers as appropriate. Reviews of nonconformities are recorded and maintained.

Any employee has the authority and responsibility to stop and/or correct service nonconformities to applicable standards.

Documented processes cover identification and reporting of nonconformance, parameters for correcting and/or discontinuing nonconforming service, and recording nonconformance.

Nonconforming material (medical products or supplies) is segregated, marked or tagged, and dispositioned. Nonconforming results or outcomes are recorded and evaluated. Concerned departments and employees are notified as appropriate.

Appropriate management staff determines the disposition of nonconformances. Disposition includes initiating corrective action, continued monitoring of the situation, or referral to a different authority.

8.4 Analysis of data

In order to verify the effectiveness of services provided by QPMC, controlled activities affecting the quality of service and the effective monitoring of the quality system ensure the continuous improvement of services. QPMC documents a procedure that outlines

Quality Paradigms Medical Center **ISO 9001:2000 Quality Systems Manual**	Quality Systems Manual Page 26 of 27
	Issued: Revised: Supersedes:

how data is collected and generated by measuring and monitoring activities for a variety of provided services. Data is reviewed and analyzed for:

- Effectiveness of services

- Efficiency levels of service structure

- Patient satisfaction

- Stakeholder satisfaction

- Process trends and patterns

- Characteristics of services

Analysis of data includes goal achievement indicators. The vice president of operations is charged with the responsibility of selecting suitable statistical methods and also identifying which data will be collected, analyzed, and utilized in conjunction with any continual improvement efforts.

8.5 Improvement

8.5.1 Continual improvement

QPMC maintains system-level procedures (Tier 2) that outline how the organization's quality policy, quality objectives, internal audit program, corrective/preventive action systems, and management reviews are facilitated for the development of continuous quality improvement strategies.

8.5.2 Corrective action

Corrective actions apply to causes of actual nonconformities.

QPMC maintains documented procedures for corrective and preventive action, corrective action logs, and preventive action logs.

Records of corrective action activities are maintained in accordance with procedures. These records document continual improvement activities.

The management representative or a designee is responsible to assign, track, verify, and close all preventive and corrective actions.

The appropriate manager distributes preventive and corrective actions. Corrective and preventive actions are reported to appropriate managers.

QPMC maintains a corrective action system to:

- Handle complaints

- Use appropriate information to detect, analyze, and determine root cause of nonconformities

Quality Paradigms Medical Center **ISO 9001:2000 Quality Systems Manual**	Quality Systems Manual Page 27 of 27
	Issued: Revised: Supersedes:

- Plan actions necessary to eliminate root causes of problems
- Control corrective action plans to ensure effectiveness

The following are reviewed for corrective action:

- Variance reports
- Patient rights complaints and investigation reports
- Findings from regulatory agencies
- Internal and external audit results
- Results of changes implemented in response to corrective action plans

All employees are responsible for reporting nonconformities. Managers initiate corrective action based on their analysis of nonconforming conditions. Action steps are defined and implemented to correct conditions adverse to quality.

8.5.3 Preventive Action

QPMC maintains a preventive action program to proactively address potential causes of nonconformities. Processes and relevant issues that may potentially cause nonconformities are identified and systematically reviewed as part of the preventive action program.

To eliminate potential causes of nonconformities in the quality system, QPMC systematically analyzes processes, trends in nonconformance, outcome measurement reports, and results of changes implemented in response to preventive action plans.

All employees have the opportunity to identify the need for a preventive action plan. Managers initiate preventive action plans as appropriate.

Procedures document the steps involved in addressing circumstances requiring preventive action. Records are maintained of all preventive action activities.

Quality Paradigms Medical Center **Quality Systems Procedure**	Control of Documents	
	Doc. No. **4.2.3**	Rev. Date:
		Page 1 of 7

Quality Paradigms Medical Center

Quality System Procedure 4.2.3

Control of Documents

Approved: _____

        VP Operations

Change Record

Date	Responsible Person	Description of Change
	Name	Initial Release

Distribution List

(list the departments that receive controlled copies)

Quality Paradigms Medical Center **Quality Systems Procedure**	Control of Documents	
	Doc. No. **4.2.3**	Rev. Date:
		Page 2 of 7

1. Purpose

- To ensure that only the most recent revision of policies, procedures, and protocols are available to appropriate personnel.

- To ensure that all documents requiring changes are revised in a timely fashion and receive required approvals.

- To ensure that the quality systems manual and quality system procedures are of current issue.

- To define the method for establishing, approving, changing, maintaining, replacing, and distributing documents.

2. Scope

All internal policies, procedures, protocols, quality systems manual, quality system–level procedures, quality policy, forms, regulatory documentation, and other external documents used for performing work are controlled.

3. Responsibilities

The executive secretary oversees the control of policies, procedures, and protocols stored electronically in the Meditech database. These documents are indexed by a listing on the opening screen for each cabinet/drawer. The list includes current revision dates, ensuring access to the most recent document.

The management representative is responsible for ensuring that all controlled hard copy ISO 9001:2000 Quality System Procedures and the quality manual are revised and approved as required, notifying employees of revisions.

Department managers or directors approve newly issued and revised policies, procedures, and protocols.

Any employee can request a change to a document, but it is up to the department manager to authorize and approve changes to documents.

The HR, Infect Control, PT Safety, and Associate Health departments are responsible for all emergency and exposure manuals. This responsibility includes their location in each department and each manual's accuracy (current documents).

4. Procedure

4.1 Types of Documents

The following documents are in the document control system.

Quality Paradigms Medical Center **Quality Systems Procedure**	Control of Documents	
	Doc. No. **4.2.3**	Rev. Date:
		Page 3 of 7

Type of Document	Description
Quality Systems Manual	Quality Systems Manual describes the elements and scope of QPMC's quality management system.
Quality System Procedure	Quality System Procedures describe the implementation of the requirements of the quality management system for the entire organization. These are hard copy controlled documents.
Policies, Procedures, and Protocols	Policies, Procedures, and Protocols describe details of practice and control specific activities. These are electronic documents in Meditech. One hard copy with approval signatures is under the control of the management representative.
Forms	Forms contain quality records. They often act as work instructions that assist the user to complete a task.

4.2 Control of the Quality Systems Manual and Quality System–Level Procedures

4.2.1 Format

The quality systems manual and quality system–level procedures have a header on each page. Both have a cover page with Title, Approval, Change Record, and Distribution List. (For the quality systems manual, this is the second page, with a title page first.)

Header for Quality Systems Manual:

Quality Paradigms Medical Center **ISO 9001:2000 Quality Systems Manual**	Quality Systems Manual Page X of XX
	Issued: Revised: Supersedes:

The following process maps define controls over documents and data within the Quality Paradigms Medical Center.

Quality Paradigms Medical Center Quality Systems Procedure	Control of Documents	
	Doc. No. **4.2.3**	Rev. Date:
		Page 4 of 7

4.2.2 Procedure for Control of the Quality System Manual and Tier 2 Procedures

Any manager may suggest a revision to a document by hand-writing changes on a copy of the document and routing to the appropriate approval authority. Any suggested changes must be signed and dated. A suggested new document is presented in draft to the area manager who routes it to the approval authority.

↓

The appropriate authority is responsible to approve document or changes to document: manual approved by the administrative council and quality system procedures approved by VP Operations. When changes are not approved, the associate who submitted the suggested change is notified by e-mail.

↓

The nature of the change made is noted on the change record. The original document with original approval signatures is sent to the management representative (MR) to issue. The master is marked on each page.

↓

Quality system procedures are controlled by the index that specifies revision date. The MR must generate a new index whenever any document is changed in the system procedure manual. A new index replaces the old one when the procedure is changed out. The change record section is updated to note the nature of any change. The MR e-mails all manual holders a notice of the change.

No ← **Quality manual?** → Yes

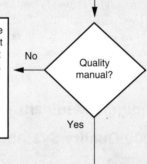

↓

MR makes a copy for each manager. Controlled copies are made with paper that has a red *controlled* watermark. Only the MR has access and authority to use this paper. For changes to documents, the MR is responsible to change out the old and remove it. One old copy may be marked *obsolete* and archived by the MR.

↓

Controlled manuals are placed in each department. The appropriate manager signs the distribution list, signifying receipt of the manual.

Quality Paradigms Medical Center Quality Systems Procedure	Control of Documents	
	Doc. No. **4.2.3**	Rev. Date:
		Page 5 of 7

4.2.3 Procedure for Control of Policies, Protocols and Procedures

Generate or revise policies, procedures, and protocols. See P&P/Admin/Policies & Procedures—Development of and P&P/Admin/Protocols—Development of.

↓

New Policy/ Procedure/Protocol?

Yes ← → No

Yes: Manager formulates document in Magic Office.

No: Document is to be revised.

E-mail to executive secretary. ← The manager e-mails the document and makes the appropriate changes.

Proofreads and verifies format, and checks spelling. ←

Correct?

No → Executive secretary makes corrections.

Yes ↓

Executive secretary will e-mail the manager a copy of the document.

↓

Manager prints a copy, signs the document, and gets appropriate additional approval signatures. (See Policy & Procedure—Development of).

↓

Document approved?

Yes ← → No

Manager e-mails the approved document to the executive secretary and places the original with approval signatures in the master binder. The manager hand-writes *obsolete* across the top of the old document in red and gives it to the executive secretary. → Executive secretary places approved documents in the correct electronic file and archives the obsolete document.

Quality Paradigms Medical Center Quality Systems Procedure	Control of Documents	
	Doc. No. **4.2.3**	Rev. Date:
		Page 6 of 7

4.4 Control of Forms

Forms at QPMC are categorized and controlled as follows:

Forms purchased from a print shop

Forms printed from Meditech's forms print and fill-in folder

Forms of external origin (state forms, forms from insurance carriers, etc.)

Forms in a single department for the department's use.

Forms are handled in accordance with Procedure 4.2.3-1 Control of Forms.

4.5 Control of Documents of External Origin

Documents of external origin are identified and indexed. Each department manager is responsible to maintain a list of external documents in use in their department.

4.6 Change Record

Quality Manual and Quality System Procedures

These documents have a change record on the first page. The date, person responsible, and nature of the change is noted. It is important to include details of the change and the page or paragraph to facilitate review.

Policies, Procedures, and Protocols

An archived copy of obsolete documents is maintained by the executive secretary as a means of establishing a change record.

Forms

The forms committee maintains a file of obsolete revisions of forms. These forms are clearly marked *obsolete* and maintained to provide a change record for future reference.

4.7 Distribution

The management representative ensures that the latest approved revisions of hard copy documents are available at the required locations, maintains the distribution list, and disposes of obsolete documents. *Obsolete* written across the top page identifies obsolete documents.

Electronic documents are only available when they have been properly approved and issued.

Quality Paradigms Medical Center **Quality Systems Procedure**	Control of Documents	
	Doc. No. **4.2.3**	Rev. Date:
		Page 7 of 7

4.8 Identification of Controlled Copy

Controlled hard copies of the quality manual and quality system procedures are indicated by a *controlled* watermark on the paper. Any copy that does not have the original watermark is uncontrolled.

For policies, procedures and protocols, the master hard copy is identified by original approval signatures and by its location in the executive secretary's master binders.

Master copies of forms are held by the management representative, with approval records from the forms committee.

4.9 Master List

The management representative is responsible to maintain the master list of quality system procedures and the master list of forms.

Policies, procedures, and protocols are indexed by department in the Meditech database.

Each department manager is responsible to maintain a list of external documents in use by their department.

4.10 Backup of Electronic Media/Data

IS is responsible for backup and storage of electronic media in accordance with the procedure so named.

5. Related Documentation

Distribution list: quality systems manual and quality system procedures index: quality systems manual and quality system procedures Meditech database

Quality Paradigms Medical Center **Quality Systems Procedure**	Control of Quality Records	
	Doc. No. **4.2.4**	Rev. Date:
		Page 1 of 4

Quality Paradigms Medical Center

Quality System Procedure 4.2.4

Control of Quality Records

Approved: _____

VP Operations

Change Record

Date	Responsible Person	Description of Change

Distribution List

All Departments

Quality Paradigms Medical Center **Quality Systems Procedure**	**Control of Quality Records**	
	Doc. No. **4.2.4**	Rev. Date:
		Page 2 of 4

1. Purpose

The purpose of records is to verify the effective operation of the quality management system. This procedure describes the activities and responsibilities associated with the handling, maintenance, and disposition of records and will ensure that records demonstrate conformance to requirements and they are legible and readily retrievable. A record is evidence that requirements were met.

2. Scope

All records required by the quality system.

3. Responsibilities

Responsibility for records is specified in the forms database or the record retention and destruction policy.

Any employee may destroy obsolete or outdated records with authorization from the appropriate manager in accordance with this procedure.

Managers are responsible to record their authorization for destruction of records.

The physical plant manager is responsible to arrange for shredding or pulping as appropriate.

4. Procedure

4.1 Identification

Records are identified on the master record control database. The access database is located on the *X* drive and viewable from all office sites. User rights are defined by levels of authority—all employees can view but only authorized designees can add to or modify the database.

4.2 Retrieval

Headings in the master record control database identify File Name, Contents Description, Location, Current/Archive, and How Filed.

These headings allow a specific record to be located.

If a hard copy record is removed from its storage location for a period of time longer than 24 hours, a file out card is placed where the file belongs identifying the record identifier, the person in possession of the record, the date it was checked out, and the date due back.

Medical records are tracked electronically in a database. Location of these records (whether stored at the office site or sent out as part of contract requirements) is tracked on a continuous basis through the database.

Quality Paradigms Medical Center Quality Systems Procedure	Control of Quality Records	
	Doc. No. **4.2.4**	Rev. Date:
		Page 3 of 4

4.3 Storage and Protection

Records are stored in file cabinets, in file boxes, or electronically. Archived files in boxes are clearly labeled to facilitate retrieval. Electronic data is backed up daily. Backups are stored off-site or in fireproof safes.

Medical records require special handling, storage, and protection (see procedure XXXX). HIPAA applies to confidentiality and privacy of records.

The mailroom is locked after business hours and staffed continuously to provide security of protected health information and other confidential correspondence.

Locked cabinets are provided for storage of confidential records. Locked storage bins are provided for documents awaiting destruction.

QPMC staff members must use password protection for their computers when left unattended. Computer monitors are positioned so that unauthorized persons cannot view the screen. Confidential information must be made unavailable in work areas when unattended by staff.

Confidential documents may be removed from an office site only with prior authorization from the appropriate manager or authorized reviewer. Documents to be mailed or delivered are marked *confidential,* taped, or otherwise packaged to ensure appropriate evidence of tampering. At no time should confidential documents be left in an area that is not secured (locked or attended).

Visitor access is controlled; visitors must register, receive a visitor badge, or be accompanied by a staff member when in work areas that contain confidential information.

4.4 Legibility

Records must be legible and written in ink, not pencil, so the information can be easily understood. Changes or corrections to records must also be legible. White-out is not acceptable. Changes must be made by striking through the old entry, writing the new information clearly in ink, and initialing the entry.

4.5 Retention

Minimum retention time is identified on the master record control database for each record. The record retention instruction defines the method for choosing an appropriate retention time.

4.6 Disposition

Records may be discarded or shredded after the minimum retention time. Records that contain financial, employee, provider, or patient information or any other documents identified as confidential are shredded. All others may be discarded. Method of disposition (shred or discard) is identified for each record on the master record control database.

Quality Paradigms Medical Center Quality Systems Procedure	Control of Quality Records	
	Doc. No. **4.2.4**	Rev. Date:
		Page 4 of 4

4.6.1 Method for shredding documents

Locked bins are provided for records identified for shredding. Employees are responsible to place such documents in the bins on a daily basis. A designee at each office is responsible for removing the documents to a secure designated area as the bins are filled. Subcontractors remove and destroy the documents from each office site per contracted schedule. Facilities management is responsible to witness the document destruction and sign the contractor's invoice.

Quality Paradigms Medical Center Quality Systems Procedure	Internal Audits	
	Doc. No. **8.2.2**	Rev. Date:
		Page 1 of 6

Quality Paradigms Medical Center

Quality System Procedure 8.2.2

Internal audits

Approved: _____
            VP Operations

Change Record

Date	Responsible Person	Description of Change

Distribution List

All Departments

Quality Paradigms Medical Center **Quality Systems Procedure**	Internal Audits	
	Doc. No. **8.2.2**	Rev. Date:
		Page 2 of 6

1. Purpose

This procedure describes the activities, responsibilities, and reporting relationships that affect the internal evaluation of QPMC's quality management system. This procedure will ensure that the quality system is maintained and that any deficiencies are addressed in a timely manner.

2. Scope

This procedure applies to the scheduling, preparation, performance, documentation, and follow-up of internal audits of QPMC's quality system, which is described by the policies and procedures covering quality related activities.

3. Responsibility

The management representative has overall responsibility for the internal audit system.

The internal audit coordinator is given specific responsibility for coordinating the internal audit program and reporting to the management representative.

The administrative assistant to the director of performance improvement inputs, tracks, and trends audit records under the direction of the internal audit coordinator.

Job descriptions for internal auditors are included in the internal auditors' job responsibilities, and performance of internal auditor responsibilities are evaluated as part of their annual performance appraisal. The management representative is responsible for including this job description in the appropriate employee files and providing input prior to an employee's performance appraisal.

The responsibility for addressing audit findings (planning and implementing corrective actions to remove and prevent nonconformance) is *not* transferred to the management representative or the audit team. It remains with the management of the audited area and ultimately with senior management at QPMC (see management responsibility section of policy manual).

After each audit activity, RAB accredited auditors are responsible for completing an RAB audit log to document the audit. Auditors are responsible for achieving and maintaining their status as RAB accredited internal auditors.

4. Procedure

4.1 Scheduling

The management representative and internal auditor coordinator (IAC) prepare a schedule of internal audits at the beginning of each calendar year indicating the month when each area of the organization included in the quality system will be audited.

Internal audit activities must be three hours in length to be credited for IRCA accreditation. This does not mean that every audit must be that long, but time for preparation and report writing for each audit activity must be included in the schedule.

Quality Paradigms Medical Center **Quality Systems Procedure**	Internal Audits	
	Doc. No. **8.2.2**	Rev. Date:
		Page 3 of 6

The sequence of areas to be audited will be based upon the flow of work through the quality system and the status and importance of the area.

Areas that form an integral part of the quality system, such as management responsibility, quality system, document control, control of quality records, and training may be examined during the course of each audit. Such audits will be designated as *regular* internal audits.

The IAC may also order additional *special* audits. The following are some reasons as to why they may be performed:

- Major revisions to existing procedures

- Changes in process, personnel, or equipment

- Findings of external auditors (customers or registrars)

- Verification of effective corrective or preventive actions

These audits may involve multiple areas, systems dealing with specific services, or other concerns.

The IAC is responsible for contacting the auditors at the beginning of each month to coordinate the selection of a specific audit date for each scheduled audit activity during that month. Audit teams are responsible for contacting the appropriate manager, agreeing on a specific schedule, and reporting the audit time and date to the IAC by e-mail. This schedule shall be finalized by the end of the first full week of each month. The IAC archives applicable e-mails in a marked cabinet.

The IAC also contacts any auditor who has not submitted audit documents on schedule and coordinates the completion of all audit activities. Failure to comply with the audit schedule without attempts to reschedule the activity results in the completion of a corrective action request by the IAC.

The IAC completes a summary report of all audit activities at the end of each month. This report is presented to the management representative and vice president of operations.

An audit planning matrix is used to schedule audits. (See Attachment 1.)

4.2 Selection and Assignment of Auditors

The IAC selects an auditor or audit team for each audit. An auditor does not have to be a QPMC employee. If an auditor is a QPMC employee, he or she must be independent of the area being audited. Auditors must have been trained in the fundamentals of auditing by an auditor that received accredited training, such as RAB and so on.

Using the internal audit schedule and previous audit reports ensures that Quality Paradigms Medical Center auditors become proficient by providing them with knowledge of this auditing procedure and experience through working on audits with qualified assessors.

Quality Paradigms Medical Center **Quality Systems Procedure**	**Internal Audits**	
	Doc. No. **8.2.2**	Rev. Date:
		Page 4 of 6

4.3 Preparation

The administrative assistant for the director of performance improvement provides the audit team with the organization's current quality manual and the current revisions of the system procedure covering the area to be audited. Audit records from prior audits of the area, if available, will also be provided.

The audit team reviews the documents provided, becoming familiar with the current system requirements and makes notes for discussion with the auditee on any portions of the documents that may be unclear.

Based on the documentation and prior audit findings, the audit team prepares questions and checklists as necessary and plans to sample records, items, and practices prior to the audit.

4.4 Audit Performance

The audit team conducts investigations and interviews based on the audit checklists. It records objective notes and observations regarding compliance or noncompliance for each requirement or question, holds a brief closing meeting with the appropriate area manager or supervisor, and leaves a copy of identified corrective actions. After completing the investigation, review the team notes taken.

The auditors are responsible for recording notes, recording findings on hard copy corrective action request (CAR) forms, and generating an audit summary. The audit record includes the completed audit summary form, copies of CARs, and any audit notes or checklists. All audit records must be completed on the day of the audit. Audit schedules include time for preparation and report writing. Auditors use their time as scheduled to complete not only interviews but also reporting activities. Reports are submitted to the internal audit coordinator within 48 hours of the activity. Reports may be submitted to the administrative assistant to the director of PI in the absence of the IAC.

After each audit activity, auditors must complete an IRCA audit log documenting the audit. Auditors are responsible for achieving and maintaining their status as IRCA accredited internal auditors.

The administrative assistant to the director of PI gives any audit records received to the IAC. After review, the IAC returns the report to the administrative assistant for input.

The administrative assistant records the CAR in the corrective action database or the corrective action log and sends a copy of the completed audit summary to the appropriate area manager and files the entire audit record in the performance improvement office.

4.5 Follow-Up

The IAC reviews all corrective actions and routes copies, as appropriate, to risk management.

Quality Paradigms **Medical Center** **Quality Systems Procedure**	**Internal Audits**	
	Doc. No. **8.2.2**	Rev. Date:
		Page 5 of 6

Follow-up actions are tracked using the corrective action process, which ensures that the effectiveness of each corrective action is verified.

CARs resulting from internal audits are verified by subsequent internal audits. The IAC schedules these as special audits.

5.0 Related Documentation

Corrective action procedure	Audit notes/checklists
Internal audit schedule	Audit summary forms
E-mails pertaining to internal audit schedules	Corrective action request forms
Internal auditor training records or credentials	Preventive action request forms
IRCA internal auditor audit logs	

Attachment 1

*QPMC Internal Audit Planning Matrix**

Department	Sect. 5	Sect. 6	7.1	7.2	7.3	7.4	7.5	7.6	8.2	8.3	8.4	8.5
Accounting			X	X		X	X		X	X	X	X
Administration	X	X	X	X		X	X		X	X	X	X
Anesthesia			X	X	X		X	X	X	X	X	X
Assoc. Health			X				X	X	X	X	X	X
Board Trustee		X	X			X	X		X	X	X	X
Billing			X				X		X	X	X	X
Case Management			X	X	X		X		X	X	X	X
Cardiac Rehab			X	X	X		X	X	X	X	X	X
Cardiac Diag.			X	X	X		X	X	X	X	X	X
Central Supply			X				X	X	X	X	X	X
Corp. Comp/RM			X				X		X	X	X	X
Dietary			X	X	X	X	X	X	X	X	X	X
EMS			X				X	X	X	X	X	X
HIM			X				X		X	X	X	X
HR		X	X				X		X	X	X	X
Infection Control			X				X		X	X	X	X
IS			X				X	X	X	X	X	X
Housekeeping			X				X		X	X	X	X
Lab			X	X			X	X	X	X	X	X
Linen			X				X		X	X	X	X
MM			X			X	X	X	X	X	X	X

continued

* Control of documents and control of records must be evaluated during all audits. Personnel training will be reviewed during all audits.

Quality Paradigms Medical Center Quality Systems Procedure	Internal Audits
	Doc. No. **8.2.2** Rev. Date:
	Page 6 of 6

continued

Department	Sect. 5	Sect. 6	7.1	7.2	7.3	7.4	7.5	7.6	8.2	8.3	8.4	8.5
Med Staff			X	X	X		X		X	X	X	X
Marketing/PR			X	X			X		X	X	X	X
Nursing Admin.			X	X	X		X	X	X	X	X	X
Nursing General			X	X	X		X	X	X	X	X	X
ED			X	X	X		X	X	X	X	X	X
OR			X	X	X		X	X	X	X	X	X
Med Surg			X	X	X		X	X	X	X	X	X
SCU			X	X	X		X	X	X	X	X	X
OB			X	X	X		X	X	X	X	X	X
Pharmacy			X	X	X	X	X	X	X	X	X	X
Reg/Central Sch.			X	X			X		X	X	X	X
Resp. Therapy			X	X	X		X	X	X	X	X	X
RAD			X	X	X		X	X	X	X	X	X
Safety			X				X	X	X	X	X	X
Social Services			X	X	X		X		X	X	X	X
Rehab			X	X	X		X	X	X	X	X	X
Physical Plant						X	X				X	
Patient Education											X	
PI											X	
Renal Dialysis								X			X	

Quality Paradigms Medical Center	Control of Nonconformity	
Quality Systems Procedure	Doc. No. **8.3**	Rev. Date:
		Page 1 of 4

Quality Paradigms Medical Center

Quality System Procedure 8.3

Control of Nonconformity

Approved: _____

  VP Operations

Change Record

Date	Responsible Person	Description of Change

Distribution List

(list the departments that receive controlled copies)

Quality Paradigms Medical Center **Quality Systems Procedure**	Control of Nonconformity	
	Doc. No. **8.3**	Rev. Date:
		Page 2 of 4

1 Purpose

To establish a process in which all nonconformities that occur within Quality Paradigms Medical Center will be reported in a timely and consistent manner. Nonconformances must be tracked and trended so that corrective action can be taken as appropriate.

2 Scope

This procedure covers all events that do not comply with current policy and procedures. Those events are termed *nonconformances*.

3 Responsibilities

The management representative reports performance improvement findings, including appropriate risk management concerns, to the vice president of operations.

The performance improvement director is responsible for tracking nonconformity findings monthly and identifying any trends in the data on a quarterly basis.

The risk/corporate compliance manager is responsible for identifying any significant risk issues on a monthly basis, tracking them quarterly, and reporting significant risk issues to the president.

The president and vice president of operations are responsible for proper communication regarding these issues.

Department managers are responsible for the following areas concerning reporting of nonconformances:

- Department implementation of all procedures, policies, protocols, and guidelines

- Collection of data

- Reporting of data

4 Procedure

Nonconformances may be identified through the following mechanisms.

Policy and Procedure	Address	Reporting method
Green Dot Safety Program	Safety	Corrective action request
Section 504 complaint proc.	Admin/Hosp	Written letter
Computer downtime	IS	IS memo
Correcting result errors	Lab Gen	Report of error
Serology quality control	Lab/Ser	Serology log book
Operating goods receipt	MM	Notes on packing slip and/or bill of lading
Merchandise return	MM	Return PO
Fetal distress	OB	Patient chart

continued

Quality Paradigms Medical Center Quality Systems Procedure	Control of Nonconformity	
	Doc. No. **8.3**	Rev. Date:
		Page 3 of 4

continued

Policy and Procedure	Address	Reporting method
Infant security abduction pol.	OB	See sentinel event
Emergency procedures	Rad/NM	Radiation Safety Board
Patient care conflict resolution (define parameters for reporting)	Nurs Admin	Patient chart
Narcotic count discrepancy	Phar	Remark column of narcotic sheet and count sheet
Peer review	Med Staff	Leadership reports, PR report
Sentinel event policy	PI	Incident report
Adverse drug reaction	Phar	Adverse Drug Reaction Report (no name in doc)
Drug recalls	Phar	Drug recall alerts from mfr. with notes and signature. Whose?
Drug reporting (quality problems)	Phar	Report to pharmacy director
Treatment of reactions to contrast materials	Rad/Rad	Radiologist's report and form # (should also be reported as ADR)
Mechanical/electrical failure	Rad/Rad	Should be reported on incident report
Serious consumer complaints	Rad/Mam	Should be attached in writing to a customer communication form
Mechanical or electrical breakdown	Rad/Gen	Should be reported via incident report
Emergency procedures	Rad/NM	Communicate to Radiation Safety Board (no form listed, refer to decontamination kit policy)
Emergency handling of radiation accident cases	Rad/NM	Communicate to Radiation Safety Board (no form listed)
Incident reporting	RM	Incident report
Customer communication	Board	Customer communication form
Hazard recognition reporting	PM	Form (preventive action?)
Medical device recalls	Safety	Manufacturer notices, recall records are stored in safety
Hospital emergency systems—handling	PM	Maintenance log
Instrument count	Surg/OR	Count record (form #)
Sharps count	Surg/OR	Count record
Sponge/sharps/instrument count	Surg/OR	Instrument, sharps, and sponge tally form (form #) Incident report
Rapid recall	Surg/Cent Proc	Written report
Death in OR	Surg/OR	Incident report

continued

Quality Paradigms Medical Center **Quality Systems Procedure**	Control of Nonconformity	
	Doc. No. **8.3**	Rev. Date:
		Page 4 of 4

continued

Policy and Procedure	Address	Reporting method
Equipment hazard operational failures	Surg/OR	Incident report: preserve instrument as is (where?)
Narcotic count discrepancy	Surg/OR	Narcotic count sheet with account of discrepancy and investigation in remarks column
Reportable infections	IC	Lab reports sent to infection control nurse and reported to infection control committee
Nosocomial infections	Phar	Patient infection forms
Drug control inspection inside pharmacy	Phar	Notes on unit inspection log
Drug control—storage, floor stock	Phar	Notes on unit inspection log
Drug control—emergency medication box	Phar	Notes on unit inspection log
Drug control—inspection outside pharmacy	Phar	Signed dated notes on unit inspection log, notifications
Physician orders or suspended medical staff	MedStaff	Notification of summary suspension (form #)

This is not an exhaustive listing. Noncompliance with any system procedure, policy, or protocol is defined as a reportable nonconformance. Unless otherwise specified, these nonconformances are reported

At the time a nonconformity is identified, it is documented on the appropriate form or report.

Department managers identify, track, trend, and analyze reported nonconformances that do not already have a clear reporting mechanism (incident reports, customer communication forms, and so on). Trends in nonconformances are reported on managers' accountability reports, and corrective action is initiated as appropriate.

5.0 Related Documentation

All policies and procedures and forms and reports as listed in section 4.

Quality System Procedure 8.5.2 Corrective Action

Quality System Procedure 8.5.3 Preventive Action

Quality System Procedure 4.2.4 Control of Quality Records

Quality Paradigms Medical Center **Quality Systems Procedure**	Corrective Action	
	Doc. No. **8.5.2**	Rev. Date:
		Page 1 of 4

Quality Paradigms Medical Center

Quality System Procedure 8.5.2

Corrective Action

Approved: _____

   VP Operations

Change Record

Date	Responsible Person	Description of Change

Distribution List

All Departments

Quality Paradigms Medical Center **Quality Systems Procedure**	Corrective Action	
	Doc. No. **8.5.2**	Rev. Date:
		Page 2 of 4

1. Purpose

These activities are the method for problem solving and continual improvement. Health Care Excel defines requirements for reviewing nonconformities, determining their causes, evaluating the need for action to prevent recurrence, determining and implementing the action, recording the results, and reviewing the corrective action taken to determine its effectiveness.

Corrective actions are appropriate to the effects of the nonconformities.

Corrective actions differ from corrections of nonconformities: a corrective action is initiated to find and resolve the *root cause* of the problem.

It is more important to choose the right indicator than to monitor every activity. A carefully chosen indicator measures all prior activities to determine the suitability and effectiveness of the procedure.

2. Scope

Companywide

3. Procedure

Nonconformities are identified and reported in accordance with Procedure 8.3 Control of Nonconformity. Supervisors review nonconformities periodically to determine the need for corrective action based on nonconformance trends and the effect of the nonconformity. Corrective action is initiated *immediately* by the supervisor or identifying employee when:

- The nonconformance impacts employee safety

- The nonconformance is a serious customer complaint

- Performance falls below the target for a quality objective

Any employee may initiate a corrective action by describing a significant nonconformance and reporting it on the form to their supervisor.

Quality Paradigms Medical Center **Quality Systems Procedure**	Corrective Action	
	Doc. No. **8.5.2**	Rev. Date:
		Page 3 of 4

Supervisors review nonconformities identified in their work area, then decide that the root cause of a nonconformance or a trend in similar nonconformities needs to be determined.

Supervisor or employee identifies an important nonconformance (impacts safety, customer complaint, or failure to meet a quality objective).

Internal auditor identifies a nonconformance during an internal audit.

↓

An employee, supervisor, or internal auditor enters a description of the discrepancy or complaint on a corrective action request (CAR), along with signature and date in the top blue section, and sends the CAR to the management representative.

↓

Management representative assigns a CAR number and designates an appropriate employee to complete the yellow section, projects a date for completion, files a copy in the CAR binder, and routes the CAR to the assigned person. CARs can be completed electronically and e-mailed. The top blue portion is now complete.

↓

Designee investigates the root cause of the discrepancy or complaint, determines an appropriate action plan, and takes action, completing the yellow section of the CAR and returning it to the management representative.

↓

Management representative schedules an internal audit to verify the effectiveness of the action taken or verifies personally, completing the bottom white section. Internal auditor returns the completed CAR to the management representative.

↓

Management representative files the completed CAR.

↓

Management representative reports to QPMC on the status of corrective actions.

Quality Paradigms Medical Center **Quality Systems Procedure**	Corrective Action	
	Doc. No. **8.5.2**	Rev. Date:
		Page 4 of 4

Reference documents

Corrective Action Request
QS-S-I-0003 Control of Nonconformance
QS-S-I-0006 Internal Audits
QS-S-I-0007 Management Review

Quality Paradigms Medical Center Quality Systems Procedure	Preventive Action	
	Doc. No. **8.5.3**	Rev. Date:
		Page 1 of 3

Quality Paradigms Medical Center

Quality System Procedure 8.5.3

Preventive Action

Approved: _____
          VP Operations

Change Record

Date	Responsible Person	Description of Change

Distribution List

All Departments

Quality Paradigms Medical Center **Quality Systems Procedure**	Preventive Action	
	Doc. No. **8.5.3**	Rev. Date:
		Page 2 of 3

1. Purpose

Preventive actions prevent potential nonconformities, providing a means for improvement that is independent from solving problems.

2. Applicability

Companywide

3. Procedure

All employees have the opportunity to identify a proposed improvement.

To eliminate potential causes of nonconformities in the quality system, the quality system management council (QSMC) analyzes:

- Processes

- Trends in nonconformance

- Outcome measurement reports

- Results of changes implemented in response to preventive action plans

An employee enters a description of the proposed improvement in the top blue section of the preventive action request (PAR) and sends it to the management representative.

↓

The management representative assigns a PAR number and reviews the proposed improvement with QSMC.

↓

QSMC determines an action plan. An action plan may be that no action will be taken at this time, or a person or team may be delegated to determine an appropriate plan of action. The yellow action plan section is completed and returned to the management representative.

↓

(A)

Quality Paradigms Medical Center **Quality Systems Procedure**	Preventive Action	
	Doc. No. **8.5.3**	Rev. Date:
		Page 3 of 3

(A)

The management representative sends a copy of the PAR with the action plan to the submitter and keeps a copy in the PAR binder.

The management representative schedules an internal audit to verify the effectiveness of the action taken or verifies personally, completing the bottom white section. The internal auditor returns the completed PAR to the management representative.

The management representative files the completed PAR.

The management representative reports to QSMC on the status of preventive actions.

Appendix C

Sample Flowcharts and Process Maps

This appendix contains a sample of various flowcharts and process maps. These samples allow a healthcare organization better understanding of the ISO 9001:2000 phrase *sequence and interaction of related processes* discussed in various chapters of this book. Additionally, these charts and maps will assist in determining how to correctly depict them as a healthcare provider begins the implementation process toward ISO 9001:2000 registration. These flowcharts and process maps alone will not be enough for the healthcare organization to meet all of the requirements of the ISO 9001:2000 standard, nor will certification be granted by simply editing these documents and using them. The charts and maps only provide a starting point for the organization.

It is highly recommended that assistance from qualified consultants be sought prior to actual creation of work flows and process maps. When seeking guidance from consultants, consider if the firm providing consultation is ISO 9001:2000 certified and if it has assisted other healthcare organizations in achieving ISO 9001:2000 certification. If additional guidance or assistance is required, please feel free to contact Bryce Carson at authors@asq.org.

General Document Control

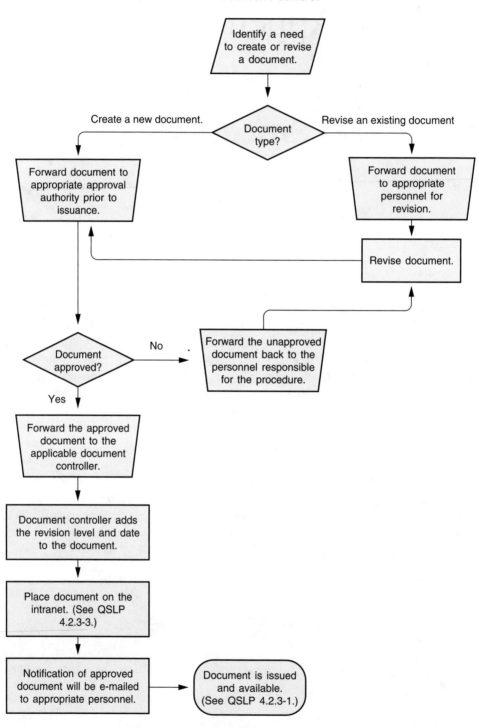

Forms Control

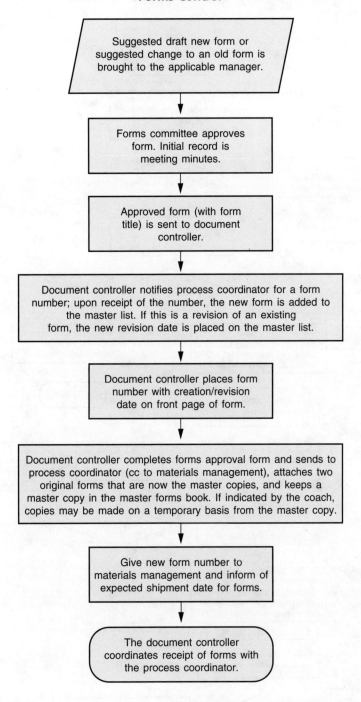

Suggested draft new form or suggested change to an old form is brought to the applicable manager.

Forms committee approves form. Initial record is meeting minutes.

Approved form (with form title) is sent to document controller.

Document controller notifies process coordinator for a form number; upon receipt of the number, the new form is added to the master list. If this is a revision of an existing form, the new revision date is placed on the master list.

Document controller places form number with creation/revision date on front page of form.

Document controller completes forms approval form and sends to process coordinator (cc to materials management), attaches two original forms that are now the master copies, and keeps a master copy in the master forms book. If indicated by the coach, copies may be made on a temporary basis from the master copy.

Give new form number to materials management and inform of expected shipment date for forms.

The document controller coordinates receipt of forms with the process coordinator.

Corrective/Preventive Action Process

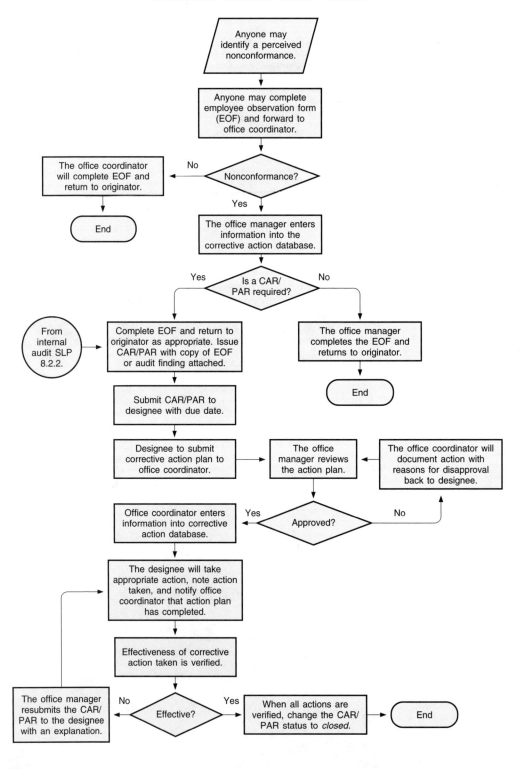

Clinical Physical Examinations Workflow

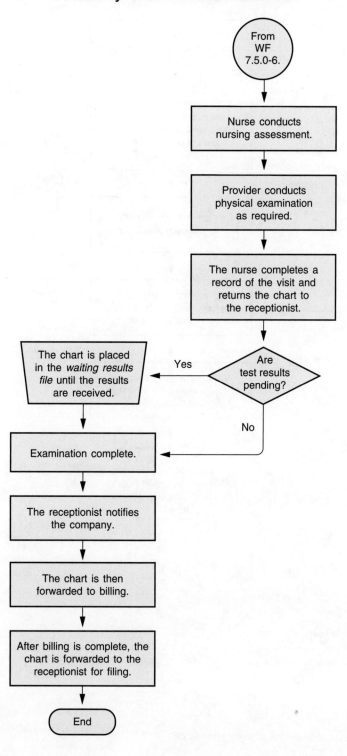

Hospital EVS Cleaning of Patient Rooms on Discharge

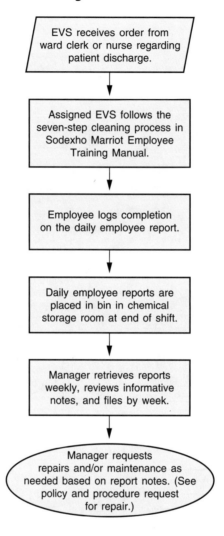

Occupational Health Clinic Basic Patient Registration Process

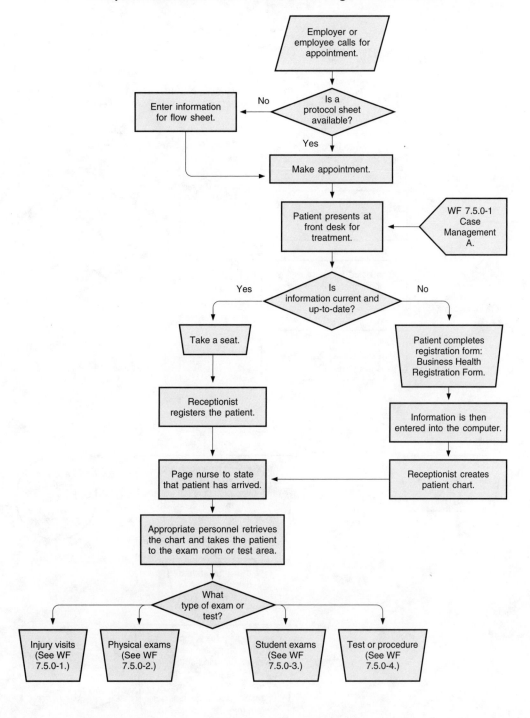

Checkout Process (Physical Discharge)

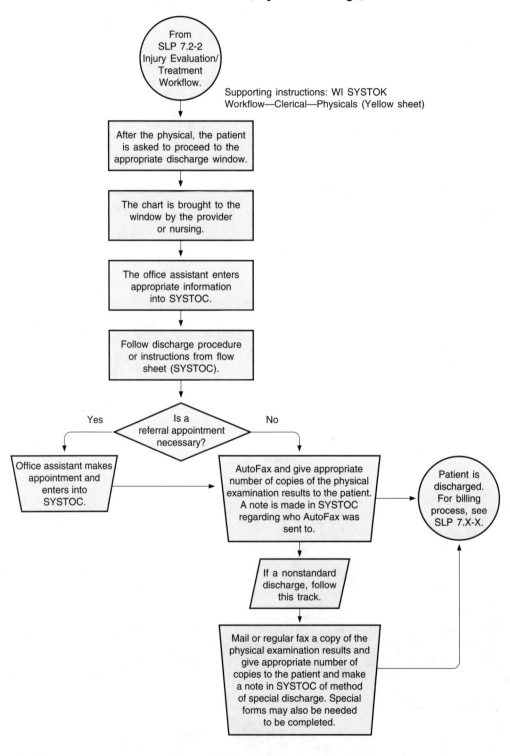

From
SLP 7.2-2
Injury Evaluation/
Treatment
Workflow.

Supporting instructions: WI SYSTOK
Workflow—Clerical—Physicals (Yellow sheet)

After the physical, the patient
is asked to proceed to the
appropriate discharge window.

The chart is brought to the
window by the provider
or nursing.

The office assistant enters
appropriate information
into SYSTOC.

Follow discharge procedure
or instructions from flow
sheet (SYSTOC).

Is a
referral appointment
necessary?

Yes

No

Office assistant makes
appointment and
enters into
SYSTOC.

AutoFax and give appropriate
number of copies of the physical
examination results to the patient.
A note is made in SYSTOC
regarding who AutoFax was
sent to.

Patient is
discharged.
For billing
process, see
SLP 7.X-X.

If a nonstandard
discharge, follow
this track.

Mail or regular fax a copy of the
physical examination results and
give appropriate number of
copies to the patient and make
a note in SYSTOC of method
of special discharge. Special
forms may also be needed
to be completed.

Hospital Sector—Appointment of Physicians

Medical secretary receives signed application.

Medical secretary requests and verifies all appropriate required information. See Physician and Other Licensed Healthcare Practitioner Appointment or Reappointment—Process Of.

Credentialing committee reviews application and supporting materials. For reappointment, the committee follows the professional and nonprofessional review standards as outlined in the medical staff bylaws.

The credentialing committee submits a written report and recommendations to the medical staff executive committee.

The medical staff executive committee recommends one of the following: accept, provisional appointment, reject, limited privileges, defer for further consideration. Recommendations and all supporting documents are sent to the board of trustees.

The board of trustees makes the final decision. If rejected, the administrator notifies the applicant via certified mail.

Injury Evaluation/Treatment Workflow

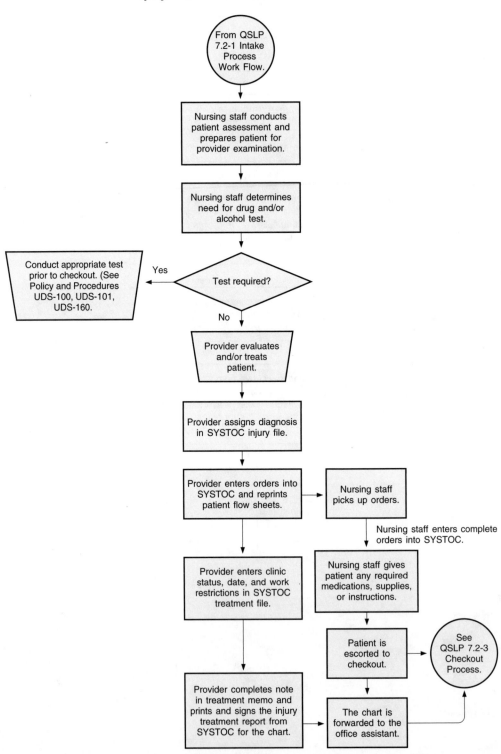

Case Management Workflow

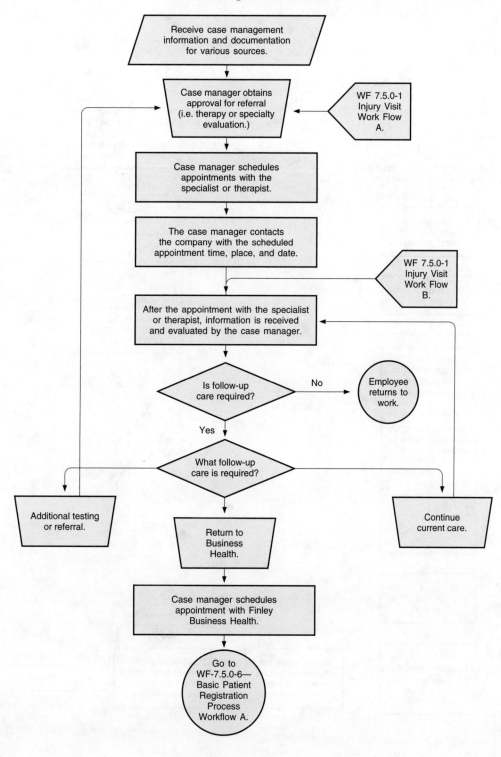

Receive case management information and documentation for various sources.

Case manager obtains approval for referral (i.e. therapy or specialty evaluation.)

WF 7.5.0-1 Injury Visit Work Flow A.

Case manager schedules appointments with the specialist or therapist.

The case manager contacts the company with the scheduled appointment time, place, and date.

WF 7.5.0-1 Injury Visit Work Flow B.

After the appointment with the specialist or therapist, information is received and evaluated by the case manager.

Is follow-up care required?

No — Employee returns to work.

Yes

What follow-up care is required?

Additional testing or referral.

Return to Business Health.

Continue current care.

Case manager schedules appointment with Finley Business Health.

Go to WF-7.5.0-6— Basic Patient Registration Process Workflow A.

Office Level Billing and Collection Process

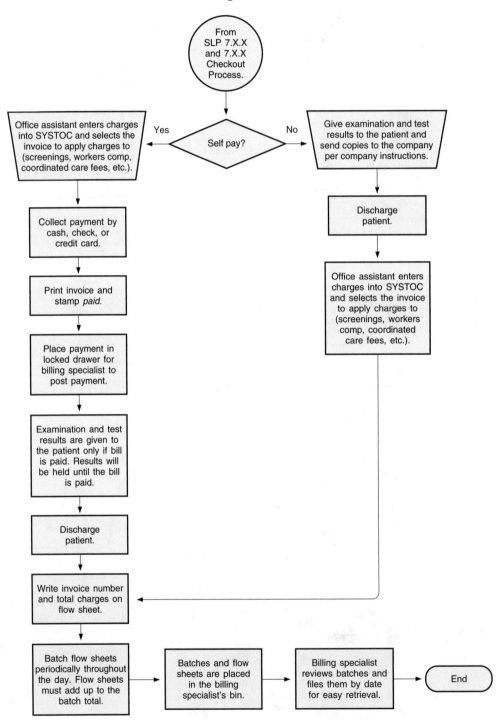

Medical Review Officer (MRO) Process

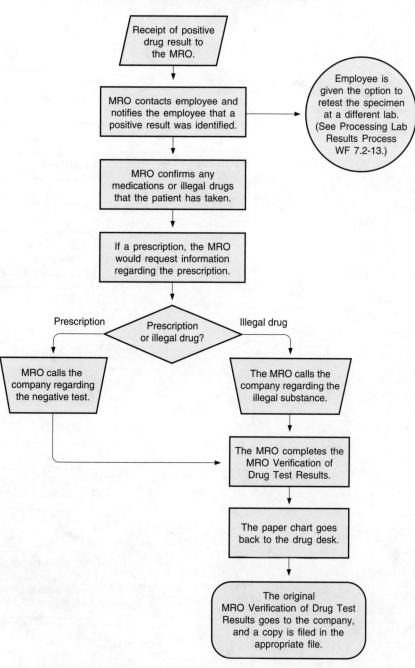

Clinical Test/Procedure Work Flow

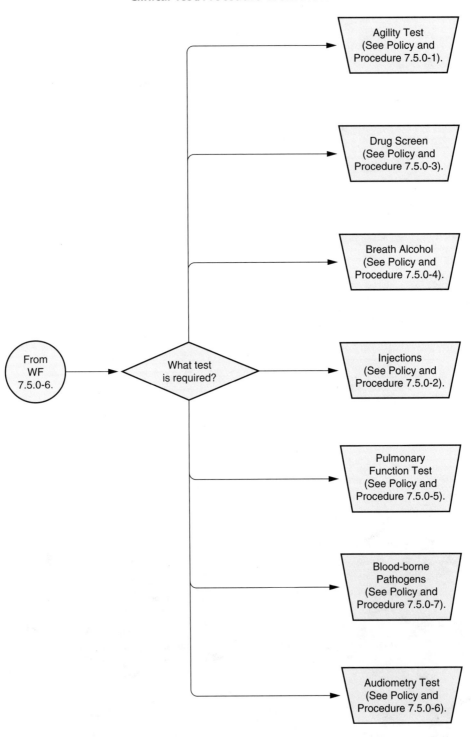

References

ANSI/ISO/ASQ Q9000-2000. *Quality management systems—Fundamentals and vocabulary.*

ANSI/ISO/ASQ Q9001-2000. *Quality management systems—Requirements.*

ANSI/ISO/ASQ Q9004-2000. *Quality management systems—Guidelines for performance improvement.*

Carson, Bryce, and Karen Brink. Aegis Group *Insight* 10, no.1 (September 2000).

Drucker, Peter F. *The Practice of Management.* New York: Harper and Row, 1967.

Hutton, Davis W. *The Change Agents' Handbook—A Survival Guide for Quality Improvement Champions.* Milwaukee: ASQC Quality Press, 1994.

Imai, Masaaki. *Kaizen—The Key to Japan's Competitive Success.* New York: McGraw-Hill/Irwin, 1986.

ISO 10013:1995. *Guidelines for Developing Quality Manuals.*

ISO 10005:1995. *Guidelines for Quality Plans.*

ISO 9000 Gets Credit for Financial Performance. http://www.asq.org/pub/qualityprogress/past/1102/21keepingCurrent1102.html, article from, www.manufacturingnews.com/news/02/0830/art1.html.

ISO 9004-4:1993. *Quality Management and Quality System Elements—Guidelines for Quality Improvement.*

Stitt, John. *Managing for Excellence—A Systematic and Holistic Analysis of the Process of Quality and Productivity Improvement.* Milwaukee: ASQC Quality Press, 1990.

About the Author

B ryce E. Carson, Sr. is vice president of Quality Paradigms Training & Consulting, an ISO 9001:2000 certified management consulting firm specializing in the implementation of ISO 9001:2000 in healthcare organizations. He is a Registrar Accreditation Board quality systems lead surveyor and senior graded IATCA assessor. Bryce has assessed over 400 manufacturing and service organizations to the ISO 9000 standards as a surveyor for accredited certification bodies. He was vice president of quality programs at Kemper Registrar Services, an accredited ISO 9000 certification body. Additionally, Carson was the lead surveyor on the first three hospitals, first physician practice, and first clinic certified to the ISO 9000 standards. He has quickly become the industry sector leader in ISO 9000 implementation in the healthcare sector. His company has led more than 100 companies and numerous healthcare organizations to successful certification.

Carson is the author of *Pressure Vessels: The ASME Code Simplified* and is a contributing author to *Quality Systems Update* on issues involving ISO 9000. He also authored the book *ISO 9001:2000 in the Assisted Reproductive Therapy Clinic*.

He has been featured in *Trustee Magazine*, the *Aegis Group Newsletter,* and *AHA News* regarding issues surrounding ISO 9000 certification in healthcare organizations. Additionally, Carson has given presentations to numerous American Society for Quality sections around the United States regarding issues of ISO 9000 for healthcare. He holds degrees in industrial engineering and quality management.

Index

A

accountability, 49
administrative team, 22
American National Standards Institute (ANSI), 13
analysis of data, 82
    sample manual, 132–33
    self-assessment, 92
ANSI/ISO/ASQ Q9001-2000 requirements,
    24–25
attachments in written procedure, 37
auditor's responsibilities, 78

C

calibration, 72–73
    equipment, 54–55
certification, 86
change agents, 85
chart audits, 77
checklists, 30
communication, internal, 49–50
    sample manual, 121
communication paths, 49
communication to patient/customer, 59
competency, clinical and medical staff, 55–56
    sample manual, 122
    self-assessment, 97
compliance audits, 77
consistent pair, 15

consulting firms, 85, 107
continual improvement, 9, 68, 82–83
    process model, 2
    sample manual, 133
continuous quality improvement (CQI) plans, 47
control, 66–67
    over processes, 67
control of documents, 38–40
    external origin, 40–41
    purpose, 39
    sample manual, 115–16
    sample procedure, 135–41
    self-assessment, 95
control of monitoring and measuring devices,
    72–73
control of nonconformity, 19–20, 81–82
    sample manual, 132
    sample procedure, 152–55
    self-assessment, 96–97
control of records, 41
    sample manual, 116
    sample procedure, 142–45
    self-assessment, 92
coordinator, quality manual, 30–31
corrective action, 83–84. *See also*
    remedial action
    sample manual, 133–34
    sample procedure, 156–59
    self-assessment, 91
credentialing, 55–56
critical processes, 22

cross-functional team, 22
customer. *See* patient/customer
customer affinity diagram, 44
customer communication, 62
    sample manual, 124
customer focus, 3–4, 18, 43–45
    sample manual, 117
customer, ISO 9000 definition, 4
customer property. *See* patient/customer
    property
customer satisfaction, 4, 11, 75–76. *See also*
    patient/customer satisfaction
customer segments, 44–45
customer-related processes, 58
    sample manual, 123–24
    self-assessment, 100
customers, identifying, 44–45

D

data analysis, 82
    sample manual, 132–33
    self-assessment, 92
decision-making, factual approach, 9, 75
definitions and terminology, quality manual, 33
    sample manual, 112–13
definitions needed in written procedure, 36
delivery of materials, equipment, and lab
    specimens, sample manual, 129
departmental objectives, 57
design and development of services, 62–64
    sample manual, 124–25
    self-assessment, 100–101
    validation, 63
    verification and documentation, 63
determination of requirements, 59–61
distribution list, quality manual, 32
documentation, amount of, 34–35
documentation requirements, 33–35
    sample manual, 115
    self-assessment, 90–91
documented procedures, 23, 24
documents, 24–25
    of external origin, 40–41
    quality manual, 25–33

quality policy, goals and objectives, 25
    referenced, 40–41
documents and records, difference between, 39

E

education requirements, clinical and medical staff,
    55–56
eight keys to improvement, 2–10
Eisenhower, Dwight D., 4
electronic communication, 50
emergencies, 59
employee involvement, 53
environment of care, 55
exclusions, 15, 17
external documents, 40–41
external requirements, 61

F

flowcharts, 68–70
flowcharts, samples, 164–76
    case management workflow, 173
    checkout process, 170
    cleaning of patient rooms, 168
    clinical physical examinations workflow, 167
    clinical test/procedure workflow, 176
    corrective/preventive action process, 166
    forms control, 165
    general document control, 164
    hospital sector—appointment of
        physicians, 171
    injury evaluation/treatment workflow, 172
    medical review officer (MRO) process, 175
    office level billing and collection process, 175
    patient registration process, 169
forms control, 40
functional objectives, 57

G

general requirements, 22–23
    sample manual, 114–15

goals, organizationwide, 25
goods and services, 18, 57
grievance process, 62
guidance, 107

H

handling patients and products, 71–72
    sample manual, 128–29
hardware, 18
hazardous materials, 72
health information service, 62
healthcare service deliverables or characteristics,
    21–22
healthcare service delivery, 18, 22
healthcare system, 19
hoshin planning, 47
how-to documents, 26
    writing, 38
human resource documentation, 53–54
human resources, 53–54
    sample manual, 122

I

identification and traceability, 70, 71
    sample manual, 127–28
    self-assessment, 96
incident reports, 19
infrastructure, 54–55
    sample manual, 122
inspection, receiving or incoming, 66
Institute of Health, 60
Institute of Medicine (IOM), xvi, xvii
internal audit, 76–80
    auditor's responsibilities, 78
    conducting, 78–80
    defined, 77
    management, 79–80
    procedure, 80
    purpose, 77–78
    sample manual, 131–32
    sample procedure, 146–51
    self-assessment, 91

    workforce, 79
internal auditor training, 86
internal audits, 22, 50, 70
internal communication, 49–50
    sample manual, 121
internal requirements, 61
International Organization for Standardization
    (ISO), 13
international standard, 15
introduction, quality management
        system, 17
    quality manual, 32
    sample manual, 114
inventory rotation, 72
involvement of people, 5–6
ISO 8402, 15
ISO 9000 certification, 1
ISO 9000 series of standards,
    history, 13–15
    ISO 9000:2000, 15
    ISO 9001:2000, 15–16
    ISO 9004:2000, 15–16
    restructuring and consolidation, 14–15
ISO 9001:2000 family of standards, 15–16
    introduction, 13
    major clause titles, 16
    normative references, 17
    scope, 17
    terms and definitions, 17–20
ISO 9001:2000, process management model, 2
    quality management principles, 2–10
    quality management system requirements,
        10
ISO team, 31
ISO technical committees, 14, 15

J

Joint Commission on Accreditation of Healthcare
        Organizations (JCAHO), 55

L

leadership, 4–5, 43

leadership and quality improvement,
self-assessment, 89–94
Libby Zion case, xvi

M

management commitment, 43
sample manual, 116
management representative, 30–31, 49
appointing, 49
sample manual, 120–21
self-assessment, 90
management responsibility, 43–52
sample manual, 116–21
self-assessment, 89–90
management review, 50
input, 50–51
output, 51
records, 50, 52
sample manual, 121
self-assessment, 90
measurement, analysis and improvement, 75–84
sample manual, 131–34
self-assessment, 91–92, 96–97
measuring and monitoring of processes and
product, 80–81
sample manual, 132
medical errors, 60
cost, xvi–xvii
medical policies and procedures, 20
medical records, 20
medication errors, 19
mentored audits, 79
monitoring and measuring devices, control, 72–73
sample manual, 129–31
self-assessment, 97

N

nonconformance reports, 19
nonconformity, control, 19–20, 81–82
sample manual, 132
sample procedure, 152–55

self-assessment, 96–97
normative references, 17

O

objectives, organizationwide, 25
occurrence reports, 19
operational planning, 48
organization size and documentation, 34
organizational data, quality manual, 33

P

packaging, sample manual, 129
patient care, 71–72
sample manual, 128–29
patient/customer, 19, 70
patient/customer needs and expectations, 44, 45,
59, 60
facility unable to meet, 61
patient/customer perceptions, 75–76
patient/customer property, 19, 70–71, 72
sample manual, 128
self-assessment, 95
patient/customer requirements, 11, 20, 60–61
process, 58
review, 20
sample manual, 123–24
patient/customer satisfaction, 43–44
sample manual, 131
patient/customer segmentation, 45
patient safety, history, xvi
personnel,
competence and documentation, 35
qualifications and training, 53–54
records, 53–54
responsibilities and authority, 49
pilot audits, 79
plan–do–check–act improvement cycle, 16
plan for the provision of care, 33
planning, 45–46
operational level, 57–58
sample manual, 117–19

three levels, 75
tools, 47
planning output documents, 48
plant equipment maintenance, 54–55
policies and procedures, 34
policy deployment, 47
preservation of product, 71–72
  sample manual, 128–29
  self-assessment, 103
preventive action, 84
  sample manual, 134
  sample procedure, 160–62
  self-assessment, 92
preventive maintenance of equipment, 54, 55
privileging, 55–56
problem solving, 8
procedure method or process, 36–37
procedure writing format, 36–37
procedures, 33–34
  paragraph headings, 36–37
  rules for writing, 35–37
procedures manual, 29–30
process, 18, 68
process approach, 6–8, 57
process complexity and documentation, 35
process management, self-assessment, 100–105
process maps. *See* flowcharts
process/system audits, 76–77
processed materials, 18
processes,
  evaluated and defined, 67–68
  managing, 8
  monitoring and measuring, 80–81
  validation, 70
processes, customer-related, 58
  sample manual, 123–24
  self-assessment, 100
product, 18, 57
  monitoring and measuring, 80–81
product and service realization, 57–73
  planning, 57–58
  sample manual, 122–31
  self-assessment, 95–96, 97, 100
product, preservation, 71–72
  sample manual, 128–29

production and service provision, 66–70
proprietary information, 30
protocols, 26
  writing, 38
provision of resources, 53
  sample manual, 121
provision of service, 66–70
  sample manual, 126–29
  self-assessment, 103
purchased product, verification, 66
  sample manual, 126
  self-assessment, 102–3
purchasing,
  sample manual, 126
  self-assessment, 101–3
purchasing information, 66
  sample manual, 126
purchasing process, 64–66
  controls, 64, 66
purpose of procedure, 36
purpose statement, quality manual, 32

Q

quality management principles, 2–10
quality management system, 21–42
  sample manual, 114–16
  self-assessment, 90–91, 92, 95
quality management system, continual
    improvement, 2
quality management system planning, 48–49
  sample manual, 118–19
quality management system requirements, 10
  key purposes, 17
  organization, 25–26
quality manual, 25–33
  acceptance, 31
  collecting information, 31
  contents, 31–33
  coordinator, 30–31
  format, 29
  header formatting, 30
  preparing to write, 29–30
  reasons for having, 29

requirements, 25–26
    sample manual, 115
    self-assessment, 90–91
    separate procedures manual, 29–30
    writing, 31
quality objectives, 46, 47
    sample manual, 117–18
quality plans, 34, 37
quality policy, 46
    communicating, 45
    goals and objectives, 25
    quality manual, 32
    sample manual, 117
    self-assessment, 89
quality system infrastructure, self-assessment, 95–99
quality system level procedures and documentation, 33–35
quality system requirements, quality manual, 33

R

recall, 73
record keeping, 41
records,
    electronic, 41
    purposes, 38
    required, 38
records and documents, difference between, 39
records in written procedure, 37
records of management review, 52
referenced documents, 40–41
references or related documents to procedures, 36
Registrar Accreditation Board (RAB), 86
regulatory requirements, 68
remedial action, 22. *See also* corrective action
requirements,
    documentation, 23–42
    general, 22–23
    nonfulfillment, 19
    omitting, 15, 17
    patient/customer, 11, 20, 60–61

resource management, 53–56
    sample manual, 121
resources, adequate, 53
responsibility, authority and communication, 49
    sample manual, 119–20
    self-assessment, 89
retesting, 73
review of requirements, 59
review, record of, 59
reviews of operations, 50
revisions or amendments, quality manual, 32

S

satisfaction feedback data, 62
scope, 17, 26
    sample manual, 113–14
scope of procedure, 36
self-assessment process, 22–23
self-assessment tool, 87–106
    leadership and quality improvement, 94
    objectivity, 87
    process management, 100–105
    quality system infrastructure, 95–99
    scoring, 88, 106
sequence and interactions flowcharts, 26–28
service delivery, 18
    sample manual, 126–27
    self-assessment, 102
service industries, 57
service provision, 66–70
    sample manual, 126–29
    self-assessment, 103
service realization. *See* product and service realization
shelf life, 72
SMART organizational goals and objectives, 25, 47
software applications, 73
special process, 18
storage, medical products, 71–72
    sample manual, 129
Stovall, Jim, 5
strategic planning, 48

study of certified companies, 86
supplier relationships, mutually beneficial, 10
suppliers, evaluating, 64–66
surveys, 76
synergy, xi
system, 19
system approach to management, 8

T

table of contents, quality manual, 32
    sample manual, 110–11
terms and definitions, 17–20
title, quality manual, 33
traceability, 70, 71
    sample manual, 127–28
    self-assessment, 96
training, clinical and medical staff, 55–56
    sample manual, 122
    self-assessment, 97
training details, 30
training records, 54

transportation of patients, 71
    sample manual, 129

U

updating procedures, quality manual, 32
U.S. Department of Commerce, 13

V

validation of processes, 70
vendors, evaluating, 65–66

W

work environment, 54–55
    sample manual, 122
workforce, educating, 79
work instructions, 26, 30
    writing, 38